ADVANCING HEALTH RIGHTS AND TACKLING INEQUALITIES

Interrogating Community Development and Participatory Praxis

Anuj Kapilashrami, Neil Quinn, and Abhijit Das

T0386059

P

First published in Great Britain in 2025 by

Policy Press, an imprint of
Bristol University Press
University of Bristol
1–9 Old Park Hill
Bristol
BS2 8BB
UK
t: +44 (0)117 374 6645
e: bup-info@bristol.ac.uk

Details of international sales and distribution partners are available at policy.bristoluniversitypress.co.uk

British Library Cataloguing in Publication Data
A catalogue record for this book is available from the British Library

ISBN 978-1-4473-6139-8 hardcover
ISBN 978-1-4473-6140-4 paperback
ISBN 978-1-4473-6141-1 ePub
ISBN 978-1-4473-6142-8 ePdf

Cover design: Liam Roberts
Front cover image: Kolitha Wickramage created this sketch based on a photograph from a participatory action research session led by Professor Kapilashrami, which explored migrant workers' health and social entitlements in urban areas.
Bristol University Press and Policy Press use environmentally responsible print partners.
Printed and bound in Great Britain by CPI Group (UK) Ltd, Croydon, CR0 4YY

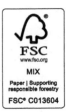

Bristol University Press' authorised representative in the European Union is:
Easy Access System Europe, Mustamäe tee 50, 10621 Tallinn, Estonia,
Email: gpsr.requests@easproject.com

Dedication

To all fellow activists committed to health justice – your courage
and determination inspire us to dream bigger and fight harder.
Together, we build a movement for change.

Contents

List of figures, boxes, and case studies

Figures

Boxes

Case Studies

Acknowledgements

We extend our sincerest thanks to all our fellow activists and scholars dedicated to health justice from whom we have had the honour of learning. Your commitment, solidarity, and intellectual companionship have fueled our passion and inspired this book, motivating us especially during these challenging times.

A special thanks to Roomi Aziz for the outstanding sketch notes, editing support, and informative illustrations that enhance our text throughout.

We are grateful to our publishers for their patience and support, as well as to the reviewers who provided invaluable feedback at various stages, particularly Maitrayee Mukhopadhyay, Tony Robertson, and Sue Laughlin. Your valuable insights have enriched our work in meaningful ways.

Lastly, we deeply appreciate the unwavering support of our families throughout this writing journey.

Anuj Kapilashrami: I would like to thank Amit for his unwavering support and for patiently listening to my dilemmas and vexations linked to global political developments that have shaped my thinking throughout this process. I am also profoundly grateful to my parents for their constant love, strength, and encouragement.

Neil Quinn: I would like to thank Katie, Remy and Cara for their constant love and support, and to Laura Paschal for generously supporting the editing of the book.

Abhijit Das: I would like to thank Jashodhara for her understanding and support.

PART I

Participation, power, and public health: historical influences and modern imperatives

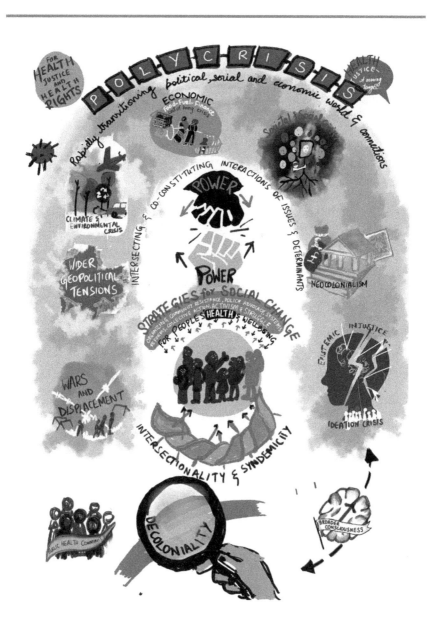

1

Introduction

This book is a synthesis of several modest live experiments that the authors were engaged in as activists and researchers committed to fostering social change through organising and collective action.

Theories about how change happens, and the role of citizens and communities in this process, lag behind the rich practice of community organising, social participation, and collective action happening around the world. Community development and social movement theories and models of participation present a valuable set of ideas that could address some of the challenges we face in attaining health goals. However, until now, these theories have not been sufficiently integrated into public health practice. They have neither been thoroughly examined from a global perspective, nor been fully incorporated into broader public health discussions, except in cases like the HIV/AIDS epidemic.

In this book, we situate practical examples of effective organising and actions from diverse geopolitical, socio-cultural and economic contexts across the Majority and Minority world, or the global South and North, integrating them within academic research. In doing so we specifically (re) examine the meanings, role, and significance of social participation and community development in advancing the right to health, tackling health inequalities, and promoting health justice. The focus is on the role of people and communities in building healthier and fair societies.

Over the past four years, the book has evolved from a mere idea into a more comprehensive and defined work. This period, which we call the 'pandemic era', has been shaped by the onset of COVID-19 and global and local efforts to address the myriad effects of the pandemic alongside rebuilding health systems and societies ravaged by it. But, most notably, this period was marked by political turmoil experienced globally. The latter include devastation of Gaza by Israeli troops, leading to instability in the Middle East, the Russian invasion and protracted violence in Ukraine, the sudden withdrawal of Western troops from Afghanistan, and the subsequent strengthening of the Taliban regime.

In response to these political events, many people around the world took part in peaceful marches and demonstrations, calling for peace, raising awareness about the health impacts of wars, and supporting humanitarian efforts. In response to the public health crises, we witnessed historic moments of widespread, grassroots resistance to protect and uphold health rights. In various countries, there were significant efforts to organise against vaccine apartheid, violations of women's rights and bodily autonomy (such as in Iran), solidarity actions addressing the housing crisis and fuel poverty, the erosion of public services (such as in the UK and Europe), and record-breaking strikes and industrial actions by health workers across Africa, Europe, and beyond, demanding improvements in health systems and working conditions.

These developments have widespread and profound implications for activism and the fight for health justice, which forms the foundation for this book. It may not be an exaggeration to say that if it were not for the pandemic and the abject handling of it in many countries, this book – and perhaps at a different time – might have turned out very differently, both in the ideas it explores and the praxis it develops around building community-led movements for change.

Why this book?

Examining the backdrop and fault lines of organising for health justice amid poly-crises

The pandemic era has taught us some crucial lessons.

One of the most significant is that the COVID-19 pandemic was not just a health crisis. It was also an economic crisis affecting both national economies and household finances; a political crisis of governance at both domestic and global levels, characterised by a mix of false claims, lack of transparency, denial, scapegoating, and populist measures. The pandemic also constituted a social and societal crisis, altering how people interacted with systems and with each other, increasing fears and anxieties, eroding trust in decision-makers, and straining the social contract between individuals and the state (The Lancet 2020). The strained contract was visible in the civic unrests and protests *against* vaccines, masks, and the scapegoating of specific communities during the pandemic.

In essence, the world is experiencing a poly-crisis.

A global **poly-crisis** occurs when crises in various interconnected global systems such as the environment, economy, migration, food security, public health, and governance – interact, leading to irreversible and harmful changes for societies and human health. The concept of poly-crisis is not new. It has been discussed in mainstream development debates for decades. Examples include the 3 F (Food, Fuel, Finance) crisis (Samuels et al 2011; Chiripanhura and Nino-Zarazua 2016) and the wicked challenges of development. Early scholarly references to poly-crisis come from complexity theorists who argued against the idea of a single threat, instead highlighting the interconnected nature of problems, crises, and uncontrollable processes that affect the planet (Lawrence et al 2024). Recently, the concept gained renewed attention at the World Economic Forum in Davos, captured in its 2024 Global Risks Report. This report paints a grim picture of the global situation, with vulnerable populations facing lethal conflicts, from Sudan to Gaza, along with extreme weather events, droughts, wildfires, and floods. It also notes the widespread societal discontent in many countries and the unprecedented polarising effects of infodemics.

These effects stem, in large part, from policy and governance failures including a lack of accountability of those in power whose actions have led to the current crises. These actions include austerity measures, the transfer of state functions to the private sector, unchecked corporate profiteering, the neglect of human rights and dignity, and the systematic weakening of public infrastructure. Commenting on the conditions that allowed COVID-19 to spread, Peter Hotez (2021) highlights the synergistic interactions of political instability and collapse (manifested as populism and political extremism), climate change, urbanisation, and displacement, shifting poverty (even within economically strong G20 countries), and the global spread of an anti-science movement, all of which have undermined the scientific and technological progress made in combating pandemics.

The research praxis surrounding health and social movements that informs this book evolved within this context. A context defined by the deeply interconnected nature of a rapidly changing political, social, and economic world.

Additionally, while there is some level of agreement among the international community on diagnosing what makes societies ill[1] – there is much less consensus on the prognosis – what to do about it. Although scholars and policymakers recognise how various global systems influence and shape each other, their responses often remain isolated and disconnected. Policy solutions tend to address one issue at a time, failing to consider the interconnected and mutually reinforcing nature of different issues, systems, and their underlying conditions. A striking example of the consequences of this siloed and fragmented approach is evident in the handling of the health of migrants and refugees. Migrants face increased disease burdens, higher risks of poor health and death, a reduced quality of life throughout their journeys, and accumulated stress in contexts they arrive in. Despite the well-documented disproportionate impact of the pandemic on migrants and refugees, the response to their health needs remains fragmented and piecemeal. The health of precarious migrants continues to be overlooked and remains peripheral to both health and labour policy agendas, which primarily focus on the health issues and working conditions of populations considered to be spatially static. Similarly, migration policies and the discourse around 'managed migration' are mainly concerned with security and regulating movement, rather than addressing the health needs of migrants.

This siloed approach to addressing global challenges is not accidental. A major obstacle to finding solutions and 'building back fairer' is a discursive or ideational crisis. Competing discourses and ideologies, along with conflicting interests of powerful actors within the governance landscape, slow down the process of change and make effective solutions difficult to achieve. These conflicts manifest in tensions between international security versus rights, growth versus post-growth and degrowth-based development, privatisation versus nationalisation of public goods, and selective versus comprehensive healthcare. These tensions were evident in policy responses to the pandemic that oscillated between protecting national economies and safeguarding public health, as well as in the debates over universal versus targeted social protection for the most affected populations.

Each of these positions reflects different ideas and claims to knowledge, which are rooted in specific ways of understanding the world (referred to as epistemes). The privileging of one set of knowledge claims or the interests of one epistemic group over others in defining health problems and solutions is a critical but missing piece in the understanding of poly-crisis. We refer to this as the ideational crisis and identify the injustice it constitutes as epistemic injustice.

Epistemic injustice refers to the concept that social and political power determines what we know and how we come to know it. This form of injustice occurs when power is used to dismiss the knowledge and perspectives of certain groups or entire nations while privileging the interests of other social or epistemic groups (Bakuni and Abimbola 2021; Besson 2022). Two specific sites and manifestations of these hegemonies are significant to public health: neoliberalism and colonial medicine.

The ideology and practice of neoliberalism has been a central driving force of economic globalisation since the late 1970s. The core principle of neoliberalism is the primacy of individual freedom and the belief that the private market is the best mechanism for allocating wealth and resources (Ife 2013). This emphasis on individual responsibility and market dominance over state provision, coupled with a shrinking state and the deregulation of trade and labour relations, challenged the post-war social democratic consensus (Springer et al 2016; Hickel 2016). The latter supported public expenditure, public borrowing, taxation, and the collective provision of public services. The rise of neoliberalism has undermined social democracy, leading nation-states to prioritise economic growth and international competitiveness over social protection. Social need got reduced to a market opportunity. Markets responded with technologies and commercial goods whose distribution has resulted in widening the gap between the rich and poor or, what some scholars refer to, making 'winners' and 'losers' from globalisation. For community development, this shift has meant the growing challenge of increased privatisation of public goods and reduced investments in welfare services, and increased disenfranchisement of marginalised communities. The financial crisis of 2008 reinforced neoliberal policies worldwide. In response to the recession, Western Europe implemented austerity measures as part of the neoliberal economic recovery strategy. These austerity policies continue to disproportionately affect deprived areas and disadvantaged communities (Beatty and Fothergill 2013), which are often the focus of community development work.

In the field of public health, another site of epistemic injustice and struggle is the dominance of the Western biomedical model. This model views health as an individual matter, determined by personal behaviours and lifestyle choices that can be measured through biological metrics and addressed through medical therapies, clinical care and pharmaceuticals.

The imposition of biomedicine was a key feature of colonialism around the world. In a recent paper, one of the authors discusses the use of pseudo-medical science by colonial powers to establish and justify white superiority and inferiority of colonised races (Mccoy et al 2024). Central to this was subjecting colonised populations to unethical medical experimentation, including vaccine and drug trials, and the erosion of rich indigenous medical systems and care practices. Christianity-led development narratives simultaneously established colonial benevolence while extending exploitative and extractive development projects.

Over the last century, these colonial practices have shaped public health, leading to the consolidation of professional power in the hands of medical doctors and the dominance of biomedical perspectives in health education, policies and decisions in global health institutions (Lassa et al 2022). The professional hegemony and social power of health professionals have become irreconcilable with those of the patients and public. This poses a central challenge for health activism. Addressing rights violations and engaging health professionals in activism requires undoing the power relations and knowledge hierarchies they are rooted in and shifting their ontological position to consider the role of politics and social environments in determining health. It also calls for recognising the central role of the community, patients, and the public in health decisions and actions.

Other barriers to advancing health rights include the altering landscape of health activism.

Changing landscape of health activism

Three key trends are prominent in this changing landscape:

On one side, contemporary activism faces a united front of nationalist, authoritarian, and neoliberal regimes that are becoming stronger, more insular, and powerful. The pandemic is witness to the rise of nationalist and populist sentiments driving state responses to global crises. For instance, major G20 nations such as the US, UK, China, India, and Russia adopted nationalist strategies for vaccine access, prioritising their own populations and engaging in bilateral vaccine sales that resulted in what is termed vaccine apartheid (Figueroa et al 2021). This trend highlights the failures of international cooperation in ensuring that tests, vaccines, and drugs reach the populations most in need. At the same time, the rise of far-right-wing ideologues and political leaders and their crackdown on human rights has shrunk the space for grassroots organisations and progressive action to advance health rights and justice. By propagating hate and misinformation, reversing rights and legal protections (for example, safe abortion, sex education) and funding, these actors have undermined the significant gains made by health rights movements. They have also triggered deep divisions in society, often along lines of identity and majoritarian politics. This environment of growing inequalities and a changing social fabric creates a significant challenge in building a social movement and advancing health rights in an environment. We explore these aspects in greater depth in this book, particularly when examining the concept of 'community' (in Chapter 2), the inclusivity of participatory development (in Chapters 3 and 4), and the rise of identity-based movements (in Chapter 5). Responding to this backlash, independent scientists and members of UN advisory groups for sexual and reproductive health recently called citizens and communities to mobilise, and to stand up for and defend health rights (Health Policy Watch 2024).

On the other side, the architecture of advocacy and resistance has never been more fragmented. This fragmentation stems from two interrelated processes. Over the past three decades, there have been significant changes in and diversification of the form and structure of civil society. One notable development is the rise of organisations that act as 'front groups' for transnational companies whose actions are harmful for people's health and the planet. These groups increase the influence of commercial actors in public policy, giving them a seat at the decision-making table. They emphasise biological and physical aspects of health, rather than the social determinants of health (Kapilashrami and Baru 2018), and advocate for individual-based and not system-based health solutions. Their influence has altered the mainstream public health discourse. Second, the shrinking space for grassroots organisations has created a stronger need for these organisations to partner with the business sector, often at the risk of depoliticising their efforts and cause (Kapilashrami and Obrien 2012). Austerity measures and funding cuts have severely limited the scope for grassroots organisations, forcing them to rely increasingly on voluntary efforts and insecure project funding tied to issue-specific grants with narrow objectives and deliverables. Large international civil society organisations (CSOs), with their advantages of scale, resources, and visibility, often partner with businesses. They crowd out grassroots organisations and bypass accountability for their 'own actions in the marketplace, including as investors, entrepreneurial fund-seekers and consumers of goods and services' (CIVICUS 2021).

Thus, civil society can act as both an extension of state and market repression and as a politically contested arena for counter-hegemonic struggle. Concomitantly, the goal of social change and health justice can be pursued either in a neoliberal sense of building civic institutions to extend states and markets, or in a Gramscian sense of building civic capacities to challenge dominant narratives, reimagine, and articulate a new vision for health and development. It is this alternative vision and reimagined approach to public and global health that the authors of this book are striving to achieve. We delve deeper into this paradox and the associated challenges in Chapters 2 and 5, while also focusing on the opportunities and actions for resistance that these conditions create.

Notwithstanding these challenges and competing standpoints, the search for alternatives and solutions to build healthy and resilient societies has never been more vigorous. A significant trend is the increasing emphasis on involving communities and placing people at the centre of planning and solutions, even though there are competing and sometimes contradictory ideas shaping this discourse.

What this book offers?

The scope of our enquiry

In this book, we bring together insights from the broader practice of community development, organising and social participation for advancing public health. The text explores the theories and models that underpin community work, participation, and health, and analyses the relationships between these concepts. It aims to deepen the understanding of how community development can promote the right to health and address health inequalities. The book introduces models of community development practice and strategies designed to improve health and well-being, while also critically examining the challenges and limitations of these approaches and their potential to drive societal change. By using examples from various international contexts, we map and identify specific areas in policy, planning, implementation, and advocacy where participation has been effective in advancing a progressive health and well-being agenda.

Our approach incorporates the critical perspectives of syndemicity and intersectionality into a decolonial framework to structure the book's content. These perspectives are implicit in issues examined, and guide the structure and strategies explored to advance health rights and equity.

Syndemicity introduces the idea that diseases occur within specific environments (physical, social, and psychological) and result from a constellation of factors, not all of which are biological. The interaction between diseases and their underlying conditions influences vulnerability and severity. This theory advocates for a broader approach to public health promotion and disease intervention (Mendenhall 2017). The concept of syndemicity helps us understand the contemporary crisis in public health, while the lens of **intersectionality** makes visible the interactions between the underlying causes of these complex challenges.

The syndemicity of diseases and the macro-level social factors or phenomena that contribute to ill health – such as climate change, disasters, conflicts, and forced displacement – necessitate a politics and form of activism that goes beyond single-issue struggles. Social movements and campaigns centred on health rights must expand their focus beyond individual patient rights to also demand systemic, institutional, and structural reforms. For example, demands for improved quality and affordability of care for individuals must be linked to efforts to challenge the growing commercialisation of healthcare services, the casualisation of labour markets, the privatisation of public goods, and holding accountable the commercial sector that manufactures ill health (such as the tobacco, alcohol, and food industries) and undermines safety nets (see Chapter 6 for commercial financing).

Intersectionality, on the other hand, is a 'conceptual lens and political tool to conceptualise and act on social inequalities' (Kapilashrami 2022, p 38). It challenges the notion that people lead single-issue lives and experience universal forms of oppression and disadvantage. Intersectionality allows us to examine how different axes of disadvantage are interconnected, making visible the links between individual lived experiences and the broader structural forces that shape them. This perspective shifts the focus from individual 'determinants' or causes of illness to the process of 'determination' of health, considering the role of broader political, economic, and environmental factors. We discuss the contribution of intersectionality and its applications in more depth in Chapters 3, 4, and 9.

Questioning the colonial epistemic gaze in community participation

In exploring the relationship between community development, participation, and health justice, this book seeks to bridge the different perspectives that have been used to theorise these fields of research and practice. We argue that the dominance of Eurocentric and Anglo-American frames of reference has created significant gaps and limitations in our current understanding and practice of community participation.

These gaps can be traced along two main fault lines, which we describe shortly.

First, a noticeable issue in mainstream scholarship on participation is its focus on privileged geopolitical contexts. It has become accepted practice for scholars and advocates, even within progressive movements, to use as reference points either political developments in the Global North (such as the UK Labour movement or the American civil rights movement) or the developmental expeditions of Northern scholars in the so-called 'Third

World'. These efforts were common during colonisation, the rebuilding of nation-states, and the subsequent era of neo-imperialism. In a review conducted to support the UK Coalition government's 'Big Society' flagship policy programme in 2010, community empowerment work was linked back to community organising efforts in the United States (Taylor-Gooby and Stoker 2011). Specifically, the review referenced Saul Alinsky's mobilisation efforts around agitation in Chicago during the 1930s and 1940s and Paulo Freire's emphasis on lived experience and critical dialogue as a foundation for transformative action. However, these references overlook the diverse grassroots struggles and activism inherent in the colonial and post-colonial histories of countries of the Global South.

The reasons for this narrow focus are acts of both omission and commission. Countries in the global South have rich histories and traditions of citizen participation in resisting occupation and building post-independence nation-states and societies. These histories are often recorded in vernacular languages, documented as handwritten monographs in library archives, and thus remain absent from mainstream scholarship. This oversight however also stems from deliberate actions to erase pre-colonial (and post-colonial) histories of community development and to discount knowledge that arises outside of the Anglo-American and Eurocentric knowledge economies.

It is during the time referenced by much of the research on community participation, that nearly a third of the world's population resided in colonies, enduring decades, if not centuries, of violence, oppression, and exploitation. Thus, community development language and models of practice need to be situated in colonial histories and sites of contestation.

The idea that people should participate in decision-making is not a new concept, as Andrea Cornwall (2006) powerfully illustrated. She traced references to participation not only in United Nations conferences and resolutions from the 1960s (such as those by the International Labour Organization and the Economic and Social Council) and amendments to the US Foreign Aid Act (in 1966 and 1973), but also to the interwar period that defined development options and led to the formation of the United Nations and Bretton Woods institutions. Cornwall argued that contemporary participation discourse often overlooks the 'policies, sentiments, and pronouncements' of the colonial past that it reflects. The philosophy of 'indirect rule', which was evident in writings from the 1920s and 1930s, utilised discourses of corruption, failed administration, and lack of accountability in colonised territories to extend governance ideas closely tied to notions of (un)civilisation and (un)development in the 'Third World'. Colonial powers invoked a sense of urgency around participation in development that made 'extraction' and exploitation morally justifiable. The historical context presented by Cornwall provides a valuable account of evolving notions of governance. Yet, these colonial ideas continue to influence current debates on 'aid effectiveness' and 'good governance'. This is evident from the disproportionate focus on LMICs in reference to corruption and transparency in governance, as well as in researching participatory development (Haldane et al 2019; Mitton et al 2011).

Referring to the practices of development agencies in the 1990s, Andrea Cornwall (2006) highlights a key aspect of epistemological bias, specifically, the way we understand and gain knowledge or how we know what we know. Cornwall effectively diagnoses the problem by noting that 'looking back has been largely confined to identifiable touchstones' (2006, p 25), that is, particularly those of the early 1970s, a period marked by enthusiasm among newly independent African states. Despite these efforts, the understanding of participation often remains confined to a Western perspective, highlighting how participation was invoked by colonial powers and their institutions – whether through indirect rule or the transfer of governance techniques in preparation for eventual self-rule. There is much less attention in mainstream literature, for reasons beyond a simple lack of scholarship, on how newly independent states and colonised nations engaged in participation and advocated for citizens' rights as they developed modern states. While Western perspectives have been critiqued for their role in determining governance functions and 'consolidating relations of rule', there has been no systematic attempt to document, understand, and incorporate the Southern practices of community-led activism and social development into mainstream community development theory. Therefore, this book seeks to address the gap caused by the epistemic injustice that overlooks the processes of colonisation and decolonisation in the Global South – processes that are crucial for understanding participation and community work.

Additionally, the book aims to address the disciplinary silos within which scholarship on community participation has developed. These silos are limited by the tendency to oversimplify (and sanitise) the complex historical processes that have shaped the relationships between the state and its citizens and to overlook the vast diversity that gives rise to these complexities. At least three broad fields of scholarship have contributed to the development of contemporary understandings of community participation and its critiques: international development studies, political science (with its focus on citizenship and rights in participatory democracies), and the more nascent field of public health and health policy. This book distils and cross-fertilises insights from these fields, identifying gaps while deepening understandings in each area.

The motivation for producing this text is partly rooted in the authors' experiences, personal politics, and reflexive praxis, which inform their engagement with the seemingly disparate epistemic worlds of academia and activism. All three authors have been deeply involved in the practice of community organising and movement building for health activism, and for women's rights. Their long-standing activism and development praxis alongside academic careers (two of the three authors located in higher education institutions) have thrown multiple challenges and dilemmas of working across epistemic divides.

The foundational ideas in this book have evolved through ongoing dialogue and critique at various points in this journey.

About this collaboration: introduction to authors' journeys

This project was conceptualised and developed through a unique partnership among authors representing diverse positionalities. Geographically dispersed and shaped by the unequal legacies of colonisation, the authors draw from a wide range of disciplinary and professional backgrounds, occupying various epistemic positions as academics, physicians, health practitioners, and human rights advocates. The decision to have authors represent these different standpoints and voices was necessary to bridge the epistemic silos that are described earlier as characterising (global) health and community development today. We hope that this approach results in ground-up writings and reflections on the key concepts discussed in this text.

However, the writing process was not always straightforward. Like the complexity and messiness of global health and development challenges and solutions, the writing does not adhere to a singular language or narrative. Instead, there are multiple perspectives on key concepts discussed reflecting views of practitioners, scholars, and advocates. It involved intense discussions and disagreements on key concepts and their application across disciplines. Community development was one such site of contestation. Authors' understanding and experience of community development practices varied based on their research and practice locations in the Global North versus the Global South. The latter generated greater scepticism towards community development work driven by donors and international agencies. The final product reveals some of these inherent tensions and potentially contested issues that remain unresolved. Readers will encounter varying degrees of criticality in the discussion of development practices in both regions. We believe this approach leads to an honest exploration of the concepts discussed in the book. In efforts to engage a diverse audience, the authors strike a balance between sharing practical examples and applications of concepts and theories and theorising from those experiences.

The authors describe their positionality in their own words as follows:

Kapilashrami: As an academic activist deeply invested in understanding the structural factors that determine health and health inequities, my work intertwines closely with activism. My early experiences with three social movements in India profoundly shaped this journey: the women's movement, the People's Health Movement (PHM), responding to the international community's failure to deliver on the promise of 'health for all', and the early sexuality rights movement against the decriminalisation of sexual identities and practices.

I began my academic journey in the UK by examining the discourse and practice of public-private partnerships in health, driven by gaps identified through health activism. During this time, significant political developments, austerity, and increasing disenfranchisement in the UK highlighted the need to strengthen health activism. This need sparked my collaboration with fellow academic activists and health professionals to revive and expand the PHM in the UK, ultimately leading to the establishment of its Scotland chapter. My engagement with deprived communities through participatory action research has also inspired similar organising efforts in neighbouring European countries facing analogous challenges.

As an academic, my research and teaching are deeply committed to addressing health inequalities and identifying transformative strategies for their reduction. Amid this work, I encountered a privileging of certain perspectives and methodologies in global health, often rooted in colonial practices. A crucial task became challenging these dominant narratives and advocating for a politics of learning and organising rooted in South-North and South-South partnerships. I employ an intersectional and decolonising perspective, actively engaging marginalised worldviews and communities in both classrooms and beyond.

Central to my work is the question of how local organising and participatory action can influence national and international policies and drive broader social change. I remain actively involved with progressive health alliances such as Health Poverty Action, PHM, and Medact, which advocate for peace, health, and social justice. These roles have been crucial for reflecting on contemporary threats to organising for health rights, building social movements, and collectively developing strategies to decolonise progressive alliances, ensuring their longevity in a volatile political environment.

Quinn: My work as a practitioner, activist, and academic has its roots in the UK. I initially trained and worked as a social worker but spent most of my career in practice as a community development worker leading a major programme focused on addressing health inequalities in East Glasgow, one of the most deprived areas in Europe. I developed several initiatives aimed at tackling mental health inequalities in partnership with marginalised communities, including people living in poverty, asylum seekers, and refugees. My work extended into the NGO sector, particularly with the Mental Health Foundation, where I contributed to various research and policy programmes. I have been involved in activism in multiple areas, including Central American solidarity, refugee rights, and the People's Health Movement. I was a member of the Oxford Guatemala Group and led the Glasgow Guatemala Group for several years, campaigning against human rights abuses in Guatemala. Over the past decade, I have played a key role in the People's Health Movement in Scotland, focusing on policy advocacy and campaigning to address health inequalities. My involvement in refugee and asylum seeker activism includes founding a local movement in Scotland to welcome refugees. As an academic, my research has focused on marginalised populations, including people with mental health problems, asylum seekers, refugees, and people experiencing homelessness. I am committed to participatory approaches and have led numerous community-based participatory research programmes. In addition to my research, I have actively influenced policy as the Co-Director (and now Founding Director) of the Centre for Health Policy at the University of Strathclyde for the past decade.

Das: My work is at the intersection of public health and social activism on the one hand, as well as practice and knowledge-making on the other. As a doctor working closely with communities in some of the most underdeveloped rural areas of North India, I witnessed the disconnect between medical knowledge and women's lived realities. The framework of 'reproductive health', which became widely used after the Cairo and Beijing Conferences, allowed me to build strong relationships with the reproductive health and women's movements. This dual engagement enabled me to critically examine public health policies and the gendered social disadvantages faced by women simultaneously. My subsequent work has focused on developing participatory mechanisms to hold the state accountable for coercive population policies and questionable family planning and maternal health programmes. At the same time, I have sought to create enabling social conditions where entire communities, particularly young men, can become allies in the broader goal of women's empowerment through their actions in both private and public spheres. This led me to explore the roles of men and masculinities and understand how privilege and intersectionality function in everyday life. Collaborating with other social activist colleagues, I realised that those working closely with communities as social innovators have unique ways of learning – methods that are intuitive, contextual, iterative, and collaborative. These 'epistemic' methods are often overlooked in formal research associated with 'development', which increasingly favours empirical, but ahistorical, atheoretical, and culturally agnostic approaches that comply with short-term project cycles. Such approaches often replicate colonial patterns. Consequently, I have been involved in developing practitioner-academic South-North collectives to promote collaborative learning.

This book extends the collaborative learning approach described by blending theory with practice and examining history and context to understand contemporary struggles and the conditions that underpin them. Through this immersive experience, we identified the need for a text that articulates the relationship between community development theory and practice and its relevance to the struggle for improving health and tackling health inequalities. The book also provides an activist's perspective on the challenges, novel approaches, and underlying conditions necessary for the realisation of health rights.

The right to health and the struggle for health justice

The concept of health as a human right and its formal adoption by member states has provided a powerful impetus for organising around health justice and emphasising equity in global health. However, as Tobin (2012) points out, the history of public health shows that societies have long recognised the necessity – whether for humanitarian, economic, or political reasons – of taking measures to protect individual health. The translation of this necessity into a formal human right to health was a much taut process and 'the product of a fragile and tentative international consensus that emerged in the wake of World War II, regarding the relationship between a state and its citizens' (Tobin 2012, p 16).

The conventional and arguably colonial discourse on human rights, as it developed in the West, was influenced by various factors. Criticisms arose about the reliance on states to uphold human rights, particularly in the context of totalitarian regimes that protected the rights of some while violating the rights of others. Other critiques focused on the exclusion of stateless people from human rights protections, the androcentric (male-centred) construction of these rights, and the perpetuation of a false dichotomy between the private and public spheres. These contestations contributed to the development of formal human rights as we know them today (Farmer et al 2013), and their interpretation within a human-rights based approach to health (Hunt 2016). A significant milestone in this process was the adoption of the Universal Declaration of Human Rights (UDHR) by the international community at the United Nations General Assembly in 1948. The UDHR outlined a series of rights that encompass both 'positive' and 'negative' liberties, including basic entitlements such as 'the right to a standard of living adequate for the health and well-being of himself and of his family, including food, clothing, housing, and medical care and necessary social services' (UDHR, Article 25), as well as a system of health protection. Additional freedoms, further defined in General Comment 14, include the right to 'control one's health and body, including sexual and reproductive freedom', and to be free from 'torture, non-consensual medical treatment, such as medical experiments and research, or forced sterilization' (General Comment No. 14, OHCHR 2000).

The UDHR's bold and holistic conception of health, along with its associated covenants, was rooted in the first formal articulation of 'the enjoyment of the highest attainable standard of health' as a fundamental right in the Constitution of the World Health Organization (WHO) in 1946. The WHO preamble defined health as 'a state of complete physical, mental, and social well-being and not merely the absence of disease or infirmity'. It emphasised that this fundamental right must be enjoyed by every human being 'without distinction of race, religion, political belief, economic or social condition', thereby acknowledging and addressing widespread social inequalities and discrimination.

However, the Cold War tensions that followed stymied these historic milestones in the international human rights movement, creating two distinct geopolitical divisions based on competing ideologies. These divisions crystallised into two international covenants (manifestos) on civil political liberties and socio-economic entitlements (Farmer et al 2013): the International Covenant on Economic, Social, and Cultural Rights (ICESCR) and the International Covenant on Civil and Political Rights (ICCPR). These covenants, while creating deep fault lines in the practice of human rights that are still evident today, together form a unified and comprehensive 'bill of rights' necessary for human development and the achievement of global health equity. In 2000, the UN Committee on Economic, Social, and Cultural Rights (CESCR), which oversees the implementation of the ICESCR, provided a more authoritative interpretation of the right to health in General Comment 14. This interpretation requires states to go beyond the preventive and curative aspects of healthcare to address the underlying determinants of health outside the healthcare sector. The ICESCR also provided a critical framework to guide health advocacy, ensuring that healthcare goods, services, and facilities are Available in adequate numbers; Accessible on financial, geographic, and non-discriminatory bases; Acceptable (meaning culturally appropriate, gender-sensitive, and ethical); and of good Quality and standards (AAAQ framework, General Comment No. 14) (CESCR 2000; de Mesquita et al 2023).

The right to health (see Figure 1.1) is considered a bridge between different aspects of human rights discourse because it is intrinsically and indivisibly linked to the realisation of other human rights (Farmer et al 2013). This is largely due to the broad conception of health endorsed in the international human rights framework, which sees timely and appropriate healthcare as necessary but not sufficient for realising the right to health (Hammonds and Ooms 2004, General Comment 14). Instead, the framework emphasises the importance of addressing the underlying social determinants of health, such as access to safe and potable water, adequate sanitation, a sufficient supply of safe food, nutrition, housing, healthy occupational and environmental conditions, and access to health-related education and information, including sexual and reproductive health. Additionally, it underscores the need for non-discrimination, transparency, and participatory processes in health-related policies and practices.

Figure 1.1: Right to health

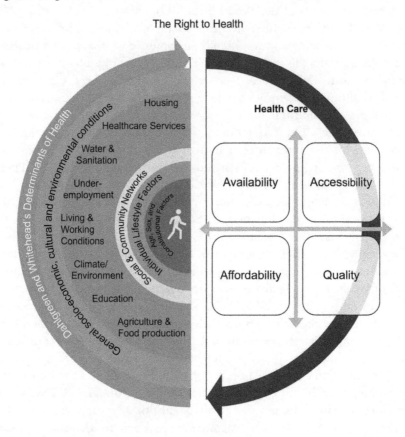

The role of communities and social participation in the struggle for health justice

The international human rights framework, along with its various instruments, provides valuable instructive guidance on the right and obligation to participate (see Box 1.1). Additionally, the primary healthcare movement made community participation a cornerstone of people-centred health systems. For example, the Declaration of Alma-Ata (1978) emphasised the 'right' and 'duty' of people to participate both individually and collectively in the planning and implementation of healthcare. It also called upon states to facilitate this participation in the 'planning, organization, operation, and control of primary health care' while educating communities about their right to participate (WHO 1978). The 2018 Declaration of Astana extended this emphasis by recognising the importance of involving individuals, communities, and civil society in the development and implementation of health-related policies and plans. Signatories of this declaration committed themselves to 'increase community ownership and contribute to the accountability of the public and private sectors so that more people can live healthier lives in environments that promote health' (WHO 2018).

Box 1.1 International Human Rights framework and instruments

UDHR Art 21: everyone has a right to participate in the governance of their country.

ICCPR Art 25: right to participate in the conduct of public affairs and to have access to public service

Gen Comment 14: notes that realising the right to health requires both individuals and groups to be entitled to participation in all government decisions affecting their health.

African Charter on Human & People's Rights, Art 13: everyone has a right to participate in governance and have equal access to the public service of their country.

These political endorsements at the international level reflect a growing consensus that community participation is not only a human right and an 'underlying determinant of realizing the right to health' (Mulumba et al 2018) but also a necessary mechanism for developing, monitoring, and delivering health services in a responsive and equitable health system. During this period, several formal mechanisms and structures evolved to enable people's participation in health, such as village health committees. These mechanisms have had varying degrees of success in achieving meaningful participation and, more importantly, in helping to realise the right to health. We examine these mechanisms in more detail in Part II.

Despite the availability of a formal human rights framework, the practice of community participation is still limited by multiple, often competing, normative frameworks.

Competing normative frameworks underpinning community participation in health

The terms participation, engagement, and involvement are frequently used interchangeably in development and health practice to describe processes by which individuals, communities, and their representatives participate in decision-making in the institutions, programmes, and environments that affect them (Florin and Wandersman 1984). The ultimate goal of these processes is the governance of public affairs. However, these terms have different origins, and their varying uses, understandings, and applications are shaped by a range of factors and forces. We map the concept of community participation across a multi-dimensional framework. The framework's axes are defined by the purpose participation is expected to serve, with one end focused on instrumental goals and the other on transformative goals; the paradigm that shapes its conception, whether participation is seen as a magic bullet or as an iterative learning process (Rifkin 1996); and the normative frameworks that underpin it, such as efficiency, effectiveness, rights, or social justice. We explore these different dimensions in greater depth in Chapter 3.

Over the years, community or social participation has served both instrumental and transformative purposes. On the instrumental side, working with communities and drawing on local knowledge has led to demonstrable improvements in health services and interventions. These improvements have made health services more effective, responsive to local needs, and more widely accepted by communities (Loewenson 2000, 2016; George et al 2015). Engaging communities in this way has also promoted values of democratic legitimacy and representation within the processes of setting health priorities (Weale et al 2016). Even in contexts where decision-making follows established formal systems and governments enjoy a high level of political legitimacy, health policy decisions can still face public resistance. Here public participation becomes essential to legitimise decisions around priorities for achieving public policy goals.

On the transformative side, certain community-led processes where people have engaged with formal systems and participated in decision-making have led to broader outcomes, such as empowering communities to claim rights and to bring the voices of often excluded groups to the forefront of planning discussions.

Empowerment, a key concept in both community development and public health, is understood as the process by which those who have been denied the ability to make strategic life choices gain that ability (Kabeer 2000, p 435). Naila Kabeer argues that the ability to exercise choice involves three interrelated components: resources (material, social, and affective or emotional assets and preconditions), agency (the power to make decisions and negotiate), and achievements (the positive changes brought about by exercising one's agency, such as improved health outcomes). Agency, in this context, is concerned with what the 'powerless' can do to shift the power relations that keep them impoverished and disenfranchised. This concept is closely tied to four dimensions of power: 'power within', which enhances self-respect and self-acceptance; 'power to', which refers to people's capacity to define their own life goals, as well as the ability to override the agency of others through exerting 'power over'. The fourth critical dimension necessary for change is collective solidarity, agency, and action, or 'power with', which refers to the ability to act together. Glenn Laverack (2005) views this as the most critical domain in the 'empowerment continuum' for achieving social and political change. It enables individuals to move from gaining control over their lives and developing their ability to assess their health needs and problems to the point where communities collectively address the deeper underlying causes that affect their health and lives (Laverack 2005, p 74). Throughout this book, we discuss lessons drawn from real-life examples of community organising and action that exemplify this fourth dimension, which aims to develop empowered communities and build solidarity.

Although not without its challenges, substantive engagement and collective action by communities have led to significant gains in making health policies and systems more responsive to people's needs, building long-term trust in public services, and, as we illustrate in this book, shifting power asymmetries at global, national, and local levels. It is this emancipatory potential of community participation – embedded in the collective struggle for health rights and justice – and our acute awareness of the limitations of an instrumental approach that define the intellectual and substantive scope of this book.

The practice of community work and development has particularly bolstered participatory initiatives and mechanisms. Community work shares many principles with the theory and practice of human rights, such as placing humanity at the core of their activities, aspiring to improve human well-being, and valuing grassroots wisdom and self-determination (Ife and Fiske 2006). The bottom-up approach, which is a core value and guiding principle of community work, explicitly recognises and seeks to redress structural oppressions. At the same time, a human rights approach offers a clear, comprehensive, and directive framework for community development practice, reminding community workers that in strengthening community, they must avoid contributing to the oppression or exclusion of people and systems beyond their immediate focus (Ife and Fiske 2006).

Despite these critical milestones, commitments, and the promise of a rights-based approach, the right to health remains marginalised in political debates and social policies around the world (Tobin 2012). It is often overlooked in the conception and implementation of programmes globally. This can be partly attributed to the dominant view of health as a commodity, a perspective reinforced by institutions like the World Bank, as well as critiques concerning the broad scope, universal applicability, and enforceability of the right to health as a legal claim (Tobin 2012; Farmer et al 2013). Paul Hunt (2016) discusses the issues of enforceability by making a distinction between three related but distinct concepts of (1) international human rights, (2) human rights-based approaches to health, and (3) the national (or domestic) right to health. Each concept has distinct implications for how the right to health is understood, promoted, and legally enforced. While the international right to health establishes a universal standard, the applicability and enforceability of health rights can be more effectively pursued through human rights-based approaches at both international and national levels.

This concurs with the differentiation made between formal and informal human rights movements (Kapilashrami et al 2015). Formal human rights movements focus on the legal frameworks that protect and promote health rights, such as access to healthcare, food security, and adequate housing. Informal human rights movements, on the other hand, involve grassroots organising with an emphasis on creating supportive empowered communities, raising awareness of entitlements, and building capacities among 'right holders' to hold 'duty bearers' accountable for not respecting or protecting these rights. This type of mobilisation requires returning to the core issue underlying human (and health) rights abuses, that is, power asymmetries. Paul Farmer and colleagues remind us that rights abuses are 'symptoms of deeper pathologies of power' (Farmer et al 2013, p xiii) that are embedded in structures of violence perpetuating poverty, inequalities in ownership and bargaining power, unequal access to education, healthcare, and food, as well as discrimination, stigma, corruption, and political instability (Farmer et al 2013, p 268).

Therefore, a key mandate of human rights informed community organising efforts is to unpack how these larger social forces constrain individual and collective agency among the disenfranchised. Equally important is the broader social change that can be achieved through such (trans)local mobilisation and the dismantling of power structures, which is critical for fulfilling rights claims (Farmer et al 2013). Throughout this book, we provide numerous examples of grassroots struggles and collective actions that illustrate how human rights-based approaches and health movements can be a powerful force for positive change.

Outline of chapters

The book uses a multi-epistemic and decolonial lens to advance our understanding of community development and participation, aiming to strengthen the practice of health justice. It is divided into three sections, each corresponding to a set of questions that assess existing theories and practices (taking stock) and chart new directions (looking forward) in the struggle for a healthier, fairer, and more just world. Throughout the book, case studies and vignettes bring together theoretical, historical, and auto-ethnographic perspectives, along with inspiring examples from practice, to provide a fresh interrogation of these fields.

Part I

The Introduction lays the foundational ideas and premise for the book. The chapter discusses how traditional global health challenges have been compounded by the multifaceted and complex crises posed by the COVID-19 pandemic and the social inequities it has exacerbated. It highlights the interconnectedness of various crises and identifies key empirical and epistemic gaps in our understanding and responses, along with their profound implications for health and development. It emphasises the importance of community participation and the need to draw insights from established fields such as community development, human rights, and public health to address these challenges through participatory praxis. The chapter also serves as a clarion call to discover new ways of working, living, and connecting in society, while protecting and promoting health rights.

The remaining chapters in this section collectively address the overarching question of how ideas of participation have evolved in the fields of public health and community development, and what contributions these ideas make in the struggle for health rights and justice. This inquiry requires an examination of the origins and genealogy of core concepts such as communities and participation, as well as the understandings of power that are central to these concepts. Chapters 2 and 3 conduct such examination.

Chapter 2 traces the long history of participatory approaches in public health (and health promotion), and their various influences, including community development. The chapter explores how pre-war colonial conquests, the post-war primary care movement, and subsequent mobilisation around development goals shaped these ideas. Focusing on the role of communities in addressing public health emergencies, the chapter examines the colonial legacies of pandemic management practices that were evident in the responses to pandemics across countries. It also looks at how civil societies responded to moral panics, infodemics, and public health restrictions. With references to both recent (COVID-19) and past pandemics, the chapter provides a powerful account of the lessons learned for strengthening community development practices in ways that are respectful of human rights and contribute to sustainable development.

Throughout this section, and particularly in Chapter 3, we emphasise the highly contested nature and meanings of key concepts like 'communities' and 'participation'. The chapter discusses the contrasting approaches and discursive underpinnings of participation, as well as their implications for practice in public health practices.

When read together, Part I underscores the importance of community participation and rights-based participatory development for achieving public health goals, answering the questions of WHY community participation is critical and what theoretical influences and development processes inform the various articulations of participation.

Part II

This part explores the objectives that people's participation serves in the struggle for health rights and justice and the pathways through which community participation and action can advance the goals of building just societies.

We identify four main strategies or pathways through which this end goal can be achieved. These strategies are interconnected and not mutually exclusive:

- Empowering the most marginalised and tackling inequities.
- Building movements for sustained advocacy and activism.
- Addressing the wider political, environmental, and commercial determinants of health.
- Holding duty bearers accountable.

Chapter 4 focuses on the first strategy: tackling unfair differences in health (health inequalities) as a key imperative for organising communities and collective action, especially among the most disadvantaged and vulnerable populations. The chapter begins by examining the nature and scale of health inequalities both across and within countries. A significant challenge in public health is that many groups, particularly those experiencing multiple deprivations and chronic precarity, are excluded from mainstream health planning and interventions. These groups are at the highest risk of poor health and bear a disproportionate burden of disease, yet they have the least access to healthcare and are often peripheral to planning and development processes. In the context of widening inequalities in health access and outcomes, this chapter explores who is excluded from mainstream development and public health practice and the limitations of participatory processes in reaching and involving these populations. Through various global case studies, it explores promising practices for engaging communities at the margins, advocating for the redistribution of power, and enhancing community ownership of health initiatives to achieve more equitable health outcomes.

Chapter 5 identifies social movements as critical conduits for achieving health rights and tackling inequalities, emphasising the vital role of health activism and advocacy, despite its often-marginal presence in public health. Building on previous work by Kapilashrami on public health advocacy, this chapter situates the experience of social movements and community organising around health rights within key debates in social movement scholarship. The latter include critical questions such as how movements arise, what they coalesce around, what distinguishes contemporary movements from older ones, and the implications of the politics of difference espoused by movements of the oppressed for health rights and justice. A central premise is that the various organising practices in the Global South offer rich lessons for community organising for health rights globally. Yet, there is a systematic neglect of Southern contributions to the theoretical understanding of social movements. Besides inspiring examples of activism to achieve public health goals, the chapter examines the case of the international People's Health Movement – one of the few broad-based transnational health movements. This *emic* account illustrates how diverse strategies of grassroots organising and global solidarity can drive systemic change for health equity.

Chapter 6 examines the third pathway, focusing on how organising communities for health and social change can influence the wider determinants of health – social, economic, political, environmental, and commercial factors outside healthcare that affect health outcomes. Through historical and contemporary case studies, such as the Cochabamba Water War and the global response to the COVID-19 pandemic, the chapter illustrates the detrimental effects of the global neoliberal economic system, policies and corporate practices on people's health and inequalities. It then explores how poor and disenfranchised communities, and social movements, have responded to these challenges. A core challenge in the struggle for health justice in pluralist societies and fragmented governance systems is ensuring accountability for health injustices and corrective action by duty bearers. The chapter calls for a united, global resistance against the intersecting crises of environment, politics, and markets to advance health rights for all.

Chapter 7 centres on this critical function of community organising and action – ensuring the accountability of state and non-state commercial actors that influence public health policy. The chapter provides examples of promising practices and mechanisms led by communities to hold duty bearers and other stakeholders accountable. In addition to specific examples where community-led accountability mechanisms have been effectively applied, the chapter discusses the limitations of such actions in the context of the complex and unstructured plurality that characterises health governance. It also examines the potential for social change by broadening the understanding of accountability processes, highlighting the 'ecosystem' of accountability and the complexities of the short and long routes adopted by activists and empowered communities.

Part III

The third part of the book is practice-oriented, structured around the tools, methods, and media available for organising communities, building movements, and fostering social change. The section begins with a reflective practitioner account of real-life advocacy efforts in India. Chapter 8 examines the role of community activism during health crises, particularly focusing on the COVID-19 pandemic. Highlighting the dual nature of state responses, oppressive and supportive, the chapter illustrates how social movements play a vital role in advancing public health, equity, and human rights, often stepping in where governmental responses fall short. It situates this discussion in a historical context of pandemics and human rights, examining how past events have shaped contemporary activism. The chapter also examines advocacy as a strategic form of activism, with a detailed look at India's long-standing fight against coercive population policies. The chapter concludes by offering strategic frameworks for effective activism, emphasising the importance of sustained collective action in achieving systemic change in health and social justice.

Chapter 9 establishes the crucial role of arts and social media in community struggles, resistance, and organising for community development and change. The chapter examines how arts and media have been used throughout the policy cycle – frame issues, build alliances, raise critical consciousness, empower communities and to support other actions for social change. By presenting examples from public health and community development, the chapter discusses the pitfalls and promises that different art forms hold in health rights movements. It also reviews the emergence and growth of digital and social media, offering case vignettes of promising practices internationally while discussing the challenges these media pose for health activism and change. The final section on participatory praxis in community health and development, specifically Participatory Action Research (PAR) discusses the core principles and role of PAR in organising communities, especially those experiencing multiple oppressions, for collective action and social change. Through specific examples, the chapter explores PAR as a significant site for contesting (and destabilising) power relations and as an alternative to traditional research approaches.

This section also questions the extent to which these tools aid or undermine political activism and organising, and what new challenges they pose for tackling health inequalities and advancing health rights in a rapidly changing world.

2

History of community participation in public health: from primary care movement to UHC

Savar is a small but bustling city about an hour's drive from Dhaka, the capital of Bangladesh. Tourists usually come to Savar to pay their respects at the National Martyrs Memorial. But between 3 and 8 December 2000, 1,450 people from 92 countries around the world gathered here to deliberate on the promise of 'Health for All by 2000' (Narayan and Schuftan 2004). They came to the campus of Gonoshasthyo Kendra, a renowned non-governmental organisation (NGO) of Bangladesh, to review the promise that the nations of the world had made in September 1978 at Alma-Ata (now Almaty) in Kazakhstan. At the International Conference on Primary Health Care in Alma-Ata, ministers, leaders, and experts from 134 countries and 67 international organisations came together and promised an acceptable level of health for all people of the world by 2000 (WHO 1978). At the 1st People's Health Assembly, in Savar, representatives of community-based organisations, social movements, trade unions, nurses, health workers, and others reviewed whether the promise made 22 years ago had indeed been fulfilled. They concluded that the 'dream never came true' and in the People's Charter for Health adopted by the delegates resolved to 'promote, support, and engage in actions that encourage people's power and control in decision-making in health at all levels' (People's Health Movement n.d.). The gathering at Savar was historic as it was a culmination of two years of active grassroots organising around health rights violations and entitlements and took the form of an organised People's Health Movement to carry forward the agenda for realising the right to health at the local, national as well as the global level.

Earlier that same year, in July 2000, during his inaugural speech at the Durban International AIDS Conference, Thabo Mbeki the President of South Africa reiterated his scepticism about the link between HIV and AIDS, saying: 'you cannot blame everything on one virus' (Fassin 2003). Infection rates from HIV/AIDS in South Africa were among the highest in the world and the activists of Treatment Action Campaign (TAC) organised a march during the conference demanding Anti-Retroviral Treatment (ART) be made freely available. In August 2001, TAC filed a case against the South African Government in the Pretoria High Court to make treatment for prevention of Mother to Child Transmission (MTCT) to mothers available outside pilot sites. On 2 July 2002, the Constitutional Court of South Africa upheld that the government indeed had a constitutional duty to provide mothers with this treatment. TAC, a campaign started by a small group of HIV-positive activists in Cape Town on 10 December 1998, had won an unprecedented victory and paved the way universal access to ARTs all over the world (Heywood 2009).

These are but two examples of how people, who are usually seen as patients or users of health services, took steps to improve or influence the way healthcare is delivered to them, and the wider social and political conditions affecting their access and improvements in health.

There is a longer and rich history of people's participation in public health; a history that is marked by paradigmatic shifts in understandings and values of participation, reflected in international commitments, subsequent global health frameworks, and the participatory practices that followed. One of the most notable shifts that continues to influence health programmes today was the move away from the aspirational comprehensive primary healthcare approach, with community empowerment at its heart, to a more selective and fragmented approach to healthcare.

In this chapter we trace these paradigmatic shifts as we explore the history and evolution of participation in the field of health, and the many contests. While charting these globally, we locate this development primarily in countries of the Global South where healthcare as we know it today is deeply influenced by colonial histories and contemporary global economic regimes.

A brief chronology of community participation in healthcare and programmes

The history of community participation in health programmes is nearly a century old. Some of the early experiences include the work of Dr B. B. Waddy, a medical officer in Ghana who trained young village men in the treatment and follow-up of river blindness, or onchocerciasis, in the 1920s and 1930s (Hardiman 1986). In pre-independent India, around the same time, F. L. Brayne a colonial officer posted in Gurgaon District, then part of rural Punjab, working closely with the rural communities introduced several public health measures including smokeless cookstoves, compost pits, soak pits, and sanitary toilets, and improved wells (Taylor 1956) as part of wider community development efforts. Subsequently the concept of engaging communities in health programming was one of the strategies outlined in the Bhore Committee report (1946) that formed the basis of health planning in independent India. After the Communist Party came to power in China, mass health programmes were introduced and one of the most successful was the campaign against schistosomiasis (Fan 2012). In the 1940s to 1970s, more local grassroots experiments emerged – where young doctors and health activists consulted local people on how they perceived their own health problems, their needs and aspirations, in the process gaining their trust and confidence. These consultations and engagement led to the development of comprehensive rural health initiatives that pioneered provision of services close to people's homes, using health teams (including community workers) in neigbourhoods, integration of services, linking medical care with provision of clean water, hygiene and nutrition, and literacy, alongside tackling discrimination (Perry and Rhode 2019). Women from communities were taught, trained, and capacitated to provide health education, improve child feeding practices, and provide basic curative care. A case in point was the Jamkhed Comprehensive Rural Health project in rural Maharashtra, India (Perry and Rhode 2019). Similar initiatives and experiences elsewhere contributed to the development of a shared Health for All by year 2000 agenda, and core principles of primary healthcare movement, adopted at Alma-Ata in 1978 (Newell 1975).

Today there are many international and global processes that identify and define a shared aspiration for all humankind like the SDGs, and its commitment to Universal Health Coverage (UHC). These commitments, prominent in the world of intergovernmental cooperation and support as we know it today, are a result of profound changes that took place after the Second World War (reflected in the changing UN membership, see Figure 2.1).

In 1945 nearly a third of the then population of the world lived in colonies of the erstwhile imperial powers like Great Britain, France, Spain, Portugal, Italy, Belgium, and Netherlands. Today, according to the United Nations, 2 million of the 7.5 billion people live in colonies. Even though the official UN figures can be contested, it undeniably constitutes a much smaller proportion. These independent nations (or erstwhile colonies) have many diversities in language, culture, topography, and histories, including colonial struggles and the distinct trajectories adopted by states that were gaining independence from colonial rule. Yet, their incorporation into the global development agenda strips off this diversity, and clusters them under homogenous classifications described by shorthand phrases of Low-and-Middle-Income Countries (LMIC) or developing countries or the global South. These differences, however, help explain how and why health-related public policy and ideas and practices of community participation have unfolded in different geopolitical contexts in distinct ways.

The history of community participation cannot therefore be understood from a single lens, most certainly not by charting developments in the warring colonial states. A dive into this history forces us to chart the colonial conquests and the birth of modern medicine and public health that resulted from it (see Figure 2.2).

Christopher Columbus' voyage across the Pacific Ocean and Vasco da Gama's discovery of a sea route around Africa to India in the 1490s opened

Figure 2.1: How the world has changed since the Second World War

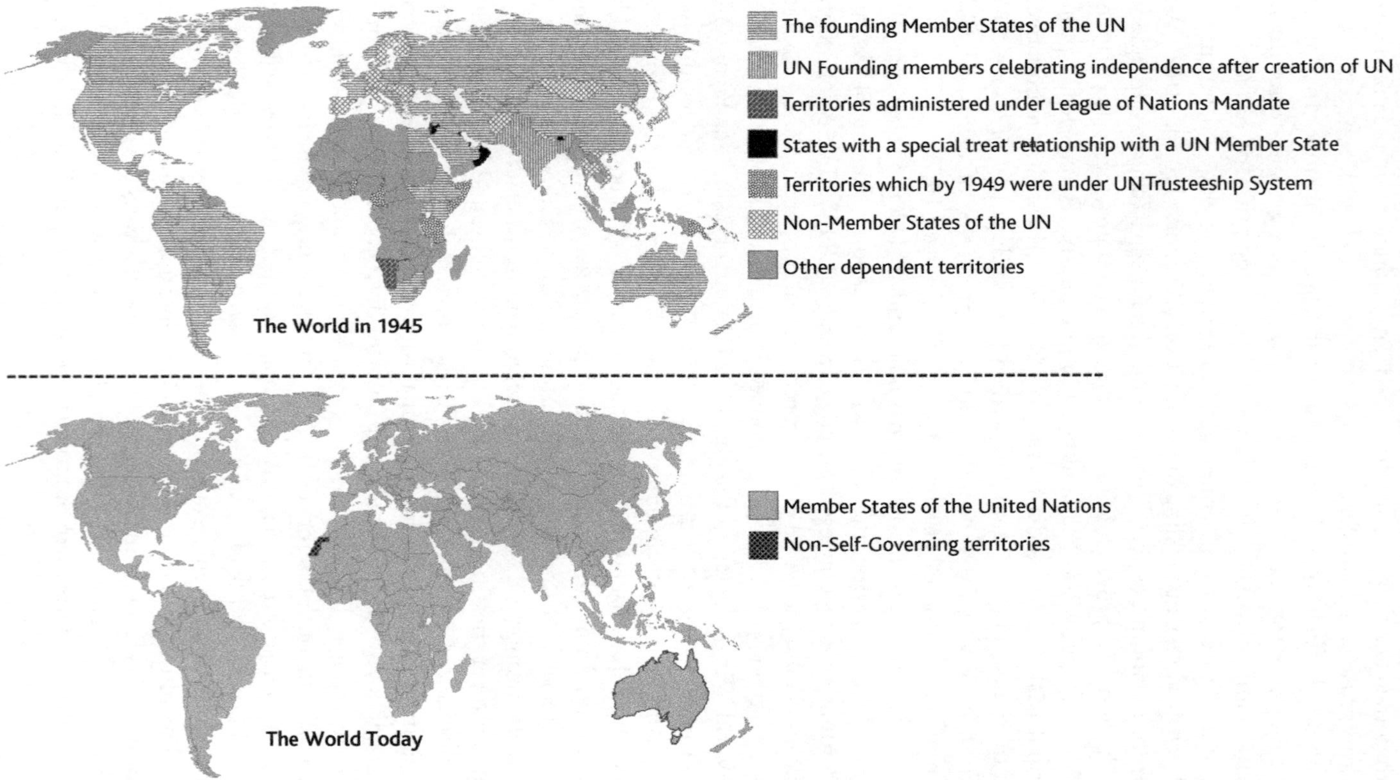

The founding Member States of the UN

UN Founding members celebrating independence after creation of UN

Territories administered under League of Nations Mandate

States with a special treat relationship with a UN Member State

Territories which by 1949 were under UN Trusteeship System

Non-Member States of the UN

Other dependent territories

The World in 1945

Member States of the United Nations

Non-Self-Governing territories

The World Today

up trade, conquest, and transfer of resources from the Americas, Africa, and Asia to Europe. This process of colonisation had far-reaching impact on the indigenous populations of these regions, a full discussion of which is beyond the scope of this chapter. One area on which colonisation had a profound impact was that of health and healthcare. The indigenous populations of the Americas were decimated by disease as well as poverty and malnutrition arising from slavery and forced labour. The role of continuing rounds of small pox epidemics in wiping out indigenous peoples in the Americas has been well documented (Ramos 2021).

Expansion of maritime trade and commerce involving coloinal ports and the resulting outbreaks and spread of pandemics (especially cholera) stimulated the first coordinated efforts of Western governments (the US and Western Europe), in the form of sanitary conferences. These focused largely on regulating and improving 'ambiguous, erratic and controversial maritime quarantine practices, land controls' (Cueto 2018, p 20) and standardising enforcement of compulsory isolation measures (Howard-Jones 1975). These conferences had the interests and priorities of the imperial European powers driving the agenda. These priorities were primarily about protection of their shores and people from diseases, the health of the economic workforce in colonies, alongside validation of the enterprise by creating a humanitarian image as well as advancing Western medicine and its prestige (through medical research outposts in Africa, Asia, and other regions of the world) (Cueto 2018). The research outposts became critical for providing the necessary research subjects, genetic material, and scientists for advancements in science.

In the early decades of colonisation, medical support from the colonising power would primarily focus on protecting the important functionaries who went abroad. It was much later that hospitals and dispensaries were established and a few doctors set up their practices or were given licences to practice in the colonies. Later, schools for training doctors and health workers were started in the colonies. There was concern about the illnesses of the sailors who returned from long voyages to the colonies in the tropics. In France, colonial medicine was taught in specialised medical schools run by the navy. The Seaman's Hospital Society was set up in London in 1817/18 for serving the needs of returning mariners and is considered a precursor of the discipline of Tropical Medicine established later by the Scottish physician Sir Patrick Manson. In the late nineteenth century the discipline of Tropical Medicine was formally established and specialised schools were set up in Liverpool and London, Lisbon, and Antwerp in the 1890s and early 1900s. Many were located in port cities and founded by shipping industrialists and became conduits of the colonial extractivist practices of international health. These continue to influence the field of global health and international development in many and significant ways.

One major interest of the colonial powers was to safeguard the health of the military and the civilian administration. Some of the developments in the growth and development of medical practice in India, considered the jewel in the crown of the British empire, provides an interesting insight. The British East India company recruited surgeons and physicians trained in Europe to serve its officers in its factories or trading posts. The position of Surgeon General was introduced as early as 1614. The Bengal Medical Services and subsequently the Madras and Bombay Medical Services were established in 1763 and 1764. To emphasise the close relationship between the practice of medicine and the military, doctors were also expected to undergo combat training. In 1858 the three separate services were unified into the Indian Medical Services. A Subordinate Medical Services was also created after 1760, comprising of Indians who were trained as dressers, compounders, and sub-assistant surgeons who were trained by the company surgeons. These 'native doctors' also had an understanding of local systems of healing and in addition to assisting the company surgeons also served the soldiers. A formal system of training such native doctors was started in 1822 through the Native Medical Institutions and this system continued for a brief period upto 1835, when the Calcutta Medical College was established to be soon followed by Medical Colleges in Madras and Bombay presidencies (Bhattacharya 2014; Saini 2016).

The British experiences from India show how with colonisation, there was not only an introduction of a new system of medicine into the colony, but also the institution of a medical hierarchy in health systems. European medical systems when introduced in colonies in Africa, Asia, and Latin America had to contend with a range of indigenous healthcare-related practices and plural healthcare systems. Many of these 'traditional' systems continue to this day. These systems are diverse, situated in distinct socio-cultural and religious contexts, and continue to be popular in some places not only because there is a lack of access to modern medicine but also because these are integrated with local belief systems and cultural practices. The arrival of 'modern' medicine established a hierarchy that relegated indigenous practices of healthcare which were now seen as backward and harmful by ruling elites. The institutionalisation of European medicine (most visible in control efforts of infectious disease outbreaks) were the early moments where the distance and disconnect of health systems from communities became visible. Thus, the disconnect and mistrust in healthcare services that we see today, and which support calls for community participation are a by-product of colonial developments of public health and medicine.

Measures to control epidemics and the spread of disease was another area leading to alienation between public authorities and the larger public in the realm of healthcare. This was true in Europe as well as in the colonies. The control of cholera, small pox, plague, and influenza epidemics through quarantine and vaccination and other 'public health' measures had elements of coercion of native populations. Such coercion and exploitation continues to this day as discussed later in Chapter 8 which traces these acts in the context of COVID-19.

Another distingushing feature and conduit of the colonial expansion was religious conversion to Christianity, which also impacted the development of public health in these contexts. Medical care, through the establishment of hospitals and dispensaries, was incorporated into Christian colonial projects, opening 'the door that the evangelist may enter in' (Calvi and Mantovanelli 2018, p 287). Medical missions became widespread in Africa and South Asia through the last quarter of the nineteenth and early twentieth centuries. Starting with a focus on spriitual salvation, the focus later shifted to healthcare as part of Christian service. In South Asia and Africa many medical missions continued to function even after independence. In Africa these missionary healthcare services received support from the national governments and played an important role in addressing key healthcare concerns like malnutrition, maternal health, and HIV/AIDS (Good 1991; Manton and Gorsky 2018). Community engagement and people's participation have emerged as key practices of many of these missionary organisations, many of whom subsequently became agents of more local grassroots organising and struggles (for example, the Catholic Health Association and the Christian Medical Association). Several organisations which emerged from such medical missionary work were represented at the People's Health Assemby at Savar. Some were even present at Alma-Ata.

After the Second World War several experiments were undertaken in the newly independent countries that laid the foundations of community participation, as enshrined in the Alma-Ata Declaration. However, the idea of community engagement in health received a pushback in the 1980s and 1990s with the rising neoliberal wave that triggered an increased participation of market forces and the gradual withdrawal of welfare functions of the state. In the 1980s and 1990s two other health-related social movements also took shape. One was the movement around HIV/AIDS and the other around women's reproductive health and rights. These are discussed later in Chapter 5. This telescopic history of the development of globally connected and at the same time disparate and contested healthcare systems is being presented to provide a context to the medical and healthcare systems that are prevalent in many Southern countries today. This history has been closely related to the political, economic, and social history of countries and continents and continues to be so. A visual timeline of these historical developments is presented in Figure 2.2.

Community health in community development

The idea of community development as we know it today has emerged on the international agenda after the Second World War and the early wave of

Figure 2.2: A simplified visual history of community participation and the fight for the right to health

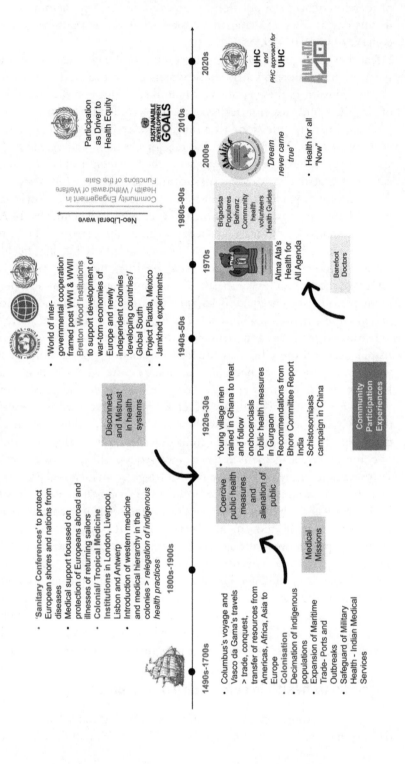

freedom from imperialism and the formation of new independent states. In the field of healthcare for poor and rural communities there were several notable experiments leading up to Alma-Ata. Among these were James Grant and C. C. Chen's work in the 1920s and 1930s in China; Sidney Kark and his colleagues' work on the pioneering Pholela model of primary healthcare, a rural Natal Province in South Africa in the 1940s and 50s; and the Khanna Study and Narangwal Study in India in the 1950s and 1960s (Tollman 1991). The Bhore Committee report of 1946 in post-independent India also recommended an integrated community-based approach to reorganising the provision of healthcare in India. Many of these models are gaining traction and getting rediscovered (Phillips 2014) as laying the foundational principles of what we understand of primary healthcare today.

A second set of experiments included a deeper engagement with the socio-economic environments that affected the health of communities. One such was Project Piaxtla, a community-based health project started in the 1966 in Sierra Madre, Mexico by David Werner, an American biologist. Based on the experiences emerging from this project, Werner wrote 'Where There is No Doctor' (Werner, Thuman, and Maxwell 1992) and 'Helping Healthworkers learn' (Werner and Bower 1982) which have served as seminal texts in the field of communty health worker training. In India, a young doctor couple, Rajnikant and Mabelle Arole, started the Comprehensive Rural Health Programme in rural Maharashtra in 1970 (Newell 1975). Illiterate women in the community were trained as health workers. The Jamkhed model not only focused on training health workers to use simple remedies but also established community-level groups where people discussed the root causes like poverty, women's status, and the caste system (Newell 1975).

The experience of the 'barefoot doctors' of China (called as such because they walked barefeet through paddy fields) in reaching communities established community health workers as a successful strategy to address the healthcare needs of rural communities. Included in the national policy in 1968 the barefoot doctors included farmers, folk healers, and others who were trained in providing preventive and curative care using a mix of traditional and modern medicine. Subsequently the approach spread across the world. In Latin America, Nicaragua the *Brigadista Populares*, or a community health volunteer, worked with communities, integrating health education with medical management. In Iran, the *Behvarz* (female frontline health worker) managed simple cases at the household-level and referred difficult cases to the hospitals or doctors. In Africa, village health worker programmes were started in many countries like Ghana, Nigeria, Tanzania, and Kenya. India introduced the Community Health Volunteer scheme and Health Guide (Prasad and Murleedharan 2007). Several such experiments around the world were compiled in the book *Health by the Community* by the

WHO and published in 1975 in preparation for the Alma-Ata Conference (Newell 1975). When the Alma-Ata Declaration was adopted in 1978, community participation practices had been successfully established as a means for encouraging poor and disadvantaged communities to engage with the development process.

In the mid-1980s the World Health Organization (WHO) adopted a new approach to health promotion that stressed increasing people's control over the determinants of their health, high-level public participation, and intersectoral cooperation (WHO 1986). The WHO-initiated Healthy Cities movement reflected this approach within urban health programmes and encouraged partnerships with nongovernmental sectors to create public policies, achieve high-level participation in community-driven projects, and, ultimately, to reduce inequities among groups (Norris and Pittman 2000).

Concurrent developments in the human rights movement bolstered the primary healthcare movement and key principles of participatory development. In 2000, through General Comment 14 of the Committee on Economic, Social and Cultural Rights, the UN clarified how the 'right to health' was to be implemented by state parties. It emphasised 'participation of the population in all health-related decision-making at the community, national and international levels' (OHCHR 2000). In the human rights-based approaches (HRBA) to development that was increasingly adopted by the UN and other development agencies from the early 2000s, communities were seen as rights-holders and development a process expected to fulfil their rights through building capacities of the 'duty bearers'. The 'good programming practices' recognised that people were to be acknowledged as key actors and not passive recipients, engaged through empowering processes where participation was both a means and a goal (HRBA Portal 2022).

The field of community development underwent some important changes in the decade of the 1990s with a series of UN-facilitated international conferences providing guidance to countries on different aspects of development. These included the United Nations Conference on Environment and Development in Rio de Janeiro in 1992, the Human Rights Conference in Vienna in 1993, the International Conference on Population and Development in Cairo in 1994, the Social Summit in Copenhagen, and the Women's Conference in Beijing. Rights and participation were included as integral principles. In 2005, a composite approach was adopted through the Millenium Development Goals (MDGs). Three of the eight goals were health focused, relating to child mortality, maternal health, and controlling diseases (AIDS, tuberculosis, and malaria). MDGs were subject to widespread criticism (Fehling, Nelson, and Venkatapuram 2013) for being less ambitious, pushing a target-oriented approach to specific health conditions, and neglecting some 'hard-fought goals' such as sexual and reproductive health and rights. In 2015 the UN adopted the 17 Sustainable Development Goals for all countries of the world. The third goal relating to health and well-being and the sixteenth goal on peaceful and inclusive societies make explicit reference to 'responsive, inclusive, participatory and representative decision-making at all levels'.

There are numerous examples from all over the world of how participatory processes enable people to engage substantially in health interventions. Some contemporary examples of how communities have come together to improve health systems and reform services at different levels are given later.

How participation affects health service delivery: state of evidence and examples from practice

Towards the end of 2012 in Madrid, Spain, thousands of citizens took to the streets opposing the proposed privatisation of health services. This started the *Marea Blanca* (White Tide), a struggle in defense of universal and free public healthcare which brought together health workers and communities from all over the country. *Marea Blanca* used *encierros* (sit-ins) and occupations of health centres and hospitals to protest against the regional government's plan to privatise healthcare (Ribera-Almandoz and Clua-Losada 2021).

In a different approach to participation, the Nhanga system was developed in Zimbabwe to enable women to have their own space. In Shona/Bantu culture, the Nhanga, which translates to 'girls' room', is a traditional round hut for girls and young women at a homestead. The Nhanga was considered a space for women's empowerment and activism, claiming it as a cultural innovation to shift harmful social norms, enhance empowering dialogue between girls and young women, and enable healing and counselling support (Gumbonzvanda, Gumbonzvanda, and Burgess 2021).

In the UK, place-based community empowerment initiatives in building collective control and improving health have gained prominence. One prominent example is the Big Lottery initiative. In this long-term (>10 years) initiative residents of 150 relatively disadvantaged areas in England receive £1 million per area to use to improve their neighbourhoods. Residents in each neighbourhood decide collectively how to use funds, within a common overall framework, developing and delivering a local plan. Governance over how the money is spent in each area rests with a resident-led partnership to enable communities to contribute to priority setting, decision-making, and plan delivery (Egan et al 2021).

In some contexts, community participation has gained wider traction and has been institutionalised through legal reforms (Arthur, Saha, and Kapilashrami 2023). Few prominent examples of such institutionalisation exist in countries such as Thailand and Brazil. Brazil adopted a new Constitution in 1988 that included the right to health within its basic framework. Soon thereafter, in 1989 Brazil introduced the SUS (Sistema Unico de Saude) or a unified health system with a vital role for citizen participation through the establishment of health councils at different levels (Martinez and Kohler 2016). These councils bring together citizens, health functionaries, and public officials to monitor the performance of programmes as well as decide on allocation of resources. This mechanism has received considerable international praise for strengthening participatory democracy. It was possible to establish health councils in Brazil because there was already a call for decentralised governance and universal healthcare through the Sanitarista movement. This broad-based social movement included both professionals and poor people and was responsible for pushing for the inclusion of health as a basic human right in the Brazilian Constitution. Emerging from the call of a social movement, the SUS covered the entire country, and health councils were established in thousands of municipalities. Brazil had one of the most remarkable improvements in health outcomes in recent times till in 2016 funding support to SUS was severely stymied (Martinez and Kohler 2016).

Thailand is one of the few countries to have successfully established community engagement as a process in UHC plans. Started in 2002, it provides essential healthcare to all citizens through three complementary health insurance schemes that are financed predominantly through tax revenue (Sumriddetchkajorn et al 2019). The legislative framework that undergirds these schemes promote participatory and responsive governance (Marshall et al 2021). The Universal Coverage Scheme includes citizens and civil society organisations in all governance and management-related committees as well as facilitation desks for patients, public disclosure of reports, 24/7 call centres, and public hearings for addressing complaints. Studies have shown that there has been a reduction in health-related expenditure among the population (Tangcharoensathien et al 2020) as well as improvement in some health outcomes (Sumriddetchkajorn et al 2019).

Several reviews have been conducted in recent years on the results of participation on health services and outcomes. A World Bank review (Mansuri and Rao 2013) on participatory development reviewed the evidence of community engagement on delivery of primary healthcare services. The review grouped the interventions aimed at community-based services into four categories: community engagement in the allocation of resources for health-related investments, in providing health-related services and information, community monitoring of healthcare providers, and decentralisation of basic health services to local governments or NGOs. The review indicated a positive impact on maternal and child health services: 30 to 80 per cent decline in infant and maternal mortality when women's groups were engaged in India and Nepal, and a significant decline in perinatal and newborn mortality in Pakistan and Bagladesh and in post neonatal mortality and mortality from diarrhoea-type diseases.

In a systematic review of impact of community participation on health services in high and upper-middle income countries (Haldane et al 2019), 49 studies were identified based on both individual- and community-level outcomes. These were organisational processes, community processes, community outcomes, health outcomes, perspectives, and empowerment. They included studies around community health, infectious and non-infectious diseases, as well as around environment and health and healthy living. Process-level outcomes like mutually agreeable organisational processes to meet a community's needs or the creation of appropriate policies and community-led priority setting were the most reported outcomes. Community-level outcomes included increased knowledge and awareness of communities, increased self-efficacy, and confidence. Health impacts were most common in non-communicable diseases interventions. The review reported both utilitarian benefits and empowerment of the disadvantaged linked to community participation.

A limitation of more instrumental approaches to community participation is linked to the purpose of engagement. This in most cases is limited to engaging people in programme implementation or monitoring; less on decision-making or priority setting. This gap is highlighted in a systematic review of evidence on community and stakeholder participation in the priority setting of publicly-funded health services and interventions (Arthur, Saha, and Kapilashrami 2023). The study led by Kapilashrami found only 27 relevant studies involving community actors in decision-making processes for defining health benefit packages, health technology assessment, and pharmaceutical coverage. While the authors identified a range of mechanisms adopted (including involvement in advisory councils, planning meetings, public hearings and focus groups, as well as other deliberative processes and public consultation methods), gaps in participation were evident. The review found that communities were engaged primarily at the data and dialogue stages of decision-making processes, with limited depth of engagement. A number of challenges, typologised as institutional/systemic, procedural, technical, and structural/normative barriers to meaningful participation, were identified in the study. The review also reports power imbalances between decision-makers and community actors and a lack of equity considerations in planning and reporting on community involvement in determining core publicly-funded health services. These findings informed the development of a technical guide led by one of the authors (Kapilashrami) commissioned by the WHO Eastern Mediterranean Regional Office of the WHO to inform community participation processes in priority setting and decision-making in countries in Eastern Mediterranean region. The guide incorporated three critical dimensions: the depth of participation, its frequency and purpose one involving, and the distinct purposes it may serve from generation of data, design, and delivery of services through to evaluation and reform. We outline the framework in Figure 2.3.

Figure 2.3: Kapilashrami's framework to guide the community participation process

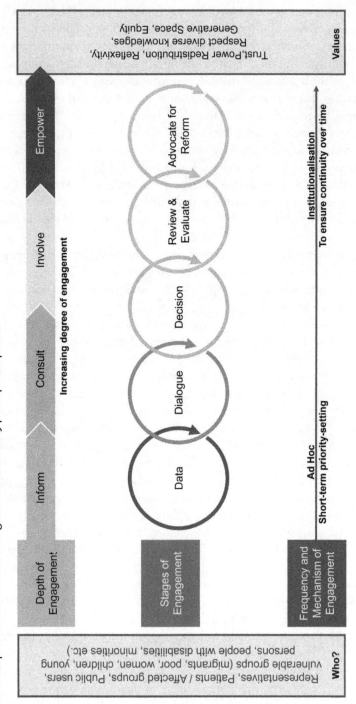

Participation at a crossroads

Even though the participation of communities has shown many benefits, it is an idea that has often been challenged. Soon after Primary Health Care was adopted, the idea was considered too idealistic and was gradually replaced by more pragmatic 'selective' primary healthcare and vertical disease-focused programme interventions. When the structural adjustment programmes started being adopted by the World Bank and the International Monetary Fund in the 1980s it called for the gradual withdrawal of the state and reduced investment in health. The focus shifted to efficiency, equity, and cost-effectiveness. The widespread adverse impact of SAPs on health are well documented (Pfeiffer and Chapman 2010; Thomson, Kentikelenis, and Stubbs 2017; Kentikelenis 2017). Later health sector reform started promoting 'user fees' in the name of participation and communities were expected to pay for services. The Bamako Initiative in 1987 formalised the introduction of user fees in public health systems in Africa, one of the poorest regions of the world (LaGuniu and Papart 2013). Two key assumptions of this approach were that communities have faith in modern medicine and that they have the money to pay. However, later experiences showed that the 'user fees' approach discriminated against the poorest, reducing access for those who need it the most (LaGunju and Papart 2013).

Mansuri and Rao (2013) in their World bank-sponsored review titled 'Localizing Development: Does Participation Work' concluded that while empowering civic groups 'may lead to good outcomes', it is not sure whether 'inducing civic empowerment is always superior to a pure market-based strategy or a strategy that strengthens the role of central bureaucrats'. The report indicates a sense of ambivalence towards externally funded and supported development projects. It found 'little evidence that induced participation builds long-lasting cohesion'. The report however recommends that participatory approaches should continue, but needed to have 'teeth', had to be supported both programmatically and financially, and needed a learning culture, backed by a strong monitoring system, and be long term.

With an increasing emphasis on participation and decentralisation, a new form of organisation – the NGO – became an important player in the community development arena. These voluntarily formed organisations are usually outside the ambit of the government and deemed as representing community interests and voices. The term 'civil society' also came into increasing usage as a 'network of groups, communities and ties that stand between the individual and the modern state' (McCowan 2023). Most formal development and health interventions as well as global health initiatives started viewing NGOs as conduits of community participation within their project frameworks. For example, in the fields of maternal health and family planning, two important areas of global concern, international NGOs

(INGOs) and coalitions, play a key role in influencing policy direction. Many of these coalitions and INGOs are led by organisations from the Global North and led by development professionals who are not personally affected by the issue.

Participation and identity

The idea of 'participation' especially in the domain of health received additional value with two movements in particular: the reproductive rights movement and the HIV/AIDS movement. These two movements brought to focus the importance of 'discrimination' and social power, and identity, rather than material conditions of deprivation and poverty, in determining health status and outcomes. The reproductive rights movement was embedded within the larger feminist articulation of women's rights, and bodily autonomy. It helped shift the conversation around family planning and population control to contraceptive choice and reproductive rights and resulted in changing the character of the global convening at the International Conference on Population and Development at Cairo in 1994. The HIV/ AIDS movement was built first by the gay community in the US who were identified as group who were affected by the disease because of their sexual preferences. Later, those who were HIV affected, including homosexuals, transgenders or sex workers who were discriminated in their own contexts, came together to define a collective 'community' and they continue to have a strong influence in the way the global as well as individual country response is shaped (WHO 2023).

Participation and the neoliberal wave

The intensifying neoliberal wave that engulfed much of the world – with rising corporate power and trade-focused economic globalisation processes – meant the states were gradually withdrawing from the welfare provisions reinstated in the post-World War context. On the one hand, this created a void that was immediately filled by complex state-market and global assemblages to deliver the functions of the state. Ranging from contracting out arrangements with the commercial private sector to service-delivering non-profit organisations, this period witnessed a burgeoning private sector filling in the financing and provisioning space and diversification of private sector financing, at both global level as well as regionally and nationally (Kapilashrami and Baru 2018). Concurrent with the growing salience of public-private partnerships in healthcare, the 'community' was extended to include other stakeholders, legitimising involvement of the commercial sector actors and industries in decision-making and priority setting in health policy.

More progressive grassroots movements on the other hand were shaping a different trajectory. Growing critiques of mainstream development and grassroots advocacy informed shifting notions of community's role in development: from passive beneficiaries and tokenistic representation to active, empowered citizens. This shift sparked the introduction of a range of innovative mechanisms of public involvement that represented a new social contract or compact between state and its citizens that served to widen healthcare access and offered a countering force to growing marketisation of healthcare. With reference to institutionalised participation introduced in the Brazil's Sistema Único de Saúde (SUS), a universal, publicly-funded, rights-based health system, Cornwall and Shankland (2008) argue that these initiatives offered 'a framework for the emergence of "regulatory partnerships" (Bloom Standing and Lloyd 2008) capable of managing the complex reality of pluralistic provision(ing)' of healthcare while ensuring that the needs of poor citizens are not marginalised.

Conclusion

Even though there is some ambivalence about the results of community participation in the larger development arena, the evidence from the field of health clearly indicates that community participation has several benefits. Today there are a whole range of stakeholders who are involved in the way healthcare services are designed and delivered. While on the one side they include patient groups, affected communities and social movements, on the other side there are powerful corporate bodies, policy makers, planners, donors, international agencies, as well as ministries of health and finance. Service providers including paramedics, nurses, and doctors are also key players. The field is replete with power assymetries, between those with the need and those who have the knowledge, skill, and resources to satisfy these needs. Participation can be seen as an important tool as well a necessary precondition that the health needs of poor, disenfranchised, and marginalised are met equitably and effectively.

3

'Communities', power, and participation: unpacking concepts from praxis

On 25 November 2020, tens of thousands of farmers from the Indian state Punjab marched towards the capital city of New Delhi demanding the repeal of a set of laws deemed detrimental to farmers. For over a year they sat on the outskirts of the city in harsh conditions, using diverse forms of protests that were met with police violence till the national government relented to some of their demands.

The idea of community is increasingly becoming vexed in a globalised world. British author David Goodheart had very simplistically divided the people of UK into two communities; the Somewheres, those who lived close to where they were originally from, and the Anywheres who are comfortable living anywhere (Goodheart 2017). He saw Brexit as a victory of the Somewheres over the Anywheres. In a very different situation People Living with HIV and AIDS (PLHA) saw themselves as a community, and pushed governments across the world for better treatment. There is a long tradition of community development practice globally, but the term community can mean several different things.

Community: a contested idea

Community is a powerful idea, with many people strongly feeling the 'loss of community' or 'loss of identity' in modern society and seeing rebuilding community structures as a priority for the future (Bauman 2001). It is simultaneously contested and problematic for the huge diversity in how communities are defined, what such diversity symbolises, and its loose reference in public and policy discourse. Over the years, governments have tended to use the term liberally in titles, speeches, and policy documents, often with little substantive meaning (Bryson and Mowbray 1981).

In its essence, community means having something in common (Twelvetrees 1991), or a group of people who are linked by common ties or bonds (Hillery 1955). Traditionally, the idea of location, spatiality, or territoriality has been an important defining characteristic for a community, with those living in the same location most likely to develop bonds with each other. These are also referred to as communities of place. However, with the development of modern globalised society, aided by the internet and technological revolution, social relations and bonds became more geographically dispersed.

Other conceptions include groups of people distinguished by shared interests or beliefs or political views (for example, human rights defenders, social activists), as well as a shared sense of identity or social position, for example, identities based on sexual and gender identity or caste.

The interest in community has been tracked back to German sociological thought in the late eighteenth and early nineteenth centuries – a time of rapid industrialisation and concerns around its impact on society. With the breakdown of traditional communities and the development of modern industrial society, a fundamental change took place in the nature of human interaction. The German sociologist, Ferdinand Tönnies (2001) made the distinction between two kinds of social relationship (Stepney and Popple 2008). One based on affection, kinship, or membership of a community, such as a family or group of friends and to describe this, Tönnies uses the German word Gemeinschaft, where people interact with a relatively small number of other people, whom they know well (Ife 2013). The other is based on a division of labour and contractual relations between isolated individuals. Tönnies referred to this society as Gesellschaft, where there are more interactions but limited to specific instrumental activities (Ife 2013).

Figure 3.1: Understanding origins, bases, and principles of community 'development'

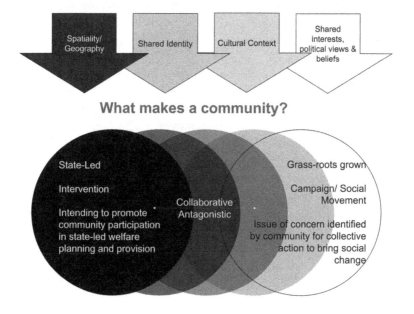

This distinction was also captured in Durkheim's definitions of organic and mechanical solidarity, which contrasted the traditional territorial communities often associated with rural life with the newer, fragmented contractual relationships that characterised industrialised urban society.

The social ties of community are contrasted with the impersonality of the state; while ideas of 'communitarianism' present it as an alternative to the state, recognising responsibilities as well as rights (Etzioni 1998). Others argue communities as mediating between state and citizen (Nisbet 1953), countering the atomistic tendencies of modern liberal societies.

Another concept that informs our understanding of community is 'social capital', which was defined as 'features of social life – networks, norms and trust' – that enable participants to act together more effectively to pursue shared objectives (Putnam 1993). Social capital provides us with a way of understanding and measuring the strength of ties and the nature of community. Strong social capital and cohesion is viewed as a positive, improving mental and physical health while acting as a buffer for harmful behaviours or risks, though it can also foster exclusion along sectarian, racial or other lines.

This is illustrated in Young and Wilmott's (1957) study of community life in Bethnal Green in London in the 1950s, which was criticised as presenting a romantic view of community life (Wilson 1980). One critic of the study, Cornwall (2008) highlighted ethnicity as determining the exclusion of black and minority ethnic residents who experienced hostility from white residents in the area. She also observed the way in which public and private accounts of community life can be at odds with each other in relation to gender, with men and women experiencing and describing notions of community differently (Cornwall 2008). This suggests that community can be more positively experienced for those with power than those who are powerless.

Important questions arise about how the community can be defined (see Figure 3.1) and what are its boundaries? Is the community geographically bound (city, neighbourhood, county; rural, urban) or defined by a common culture (defined by ethnic identity), human/health condition (parents of children with special needs)? Or bound by a shared concern and joint action, for example, climate activists, survivors of violence? There are also questions of who represents a community and its voice, whose interests prevail, who wields power and how such power determines one's chances of participating in and benefiting from community development or remaining excluded from these. For example, in community development, while working with local organisations provides the infrastructure necessary to forge relationships, not all organisations can represent the diverse voices and interests in community or reach the most disadvantaged. We examine this further when discussing ideas of participation and power.

In a nutshell, the term 'community' often assumes homogeneity, cohesiveness, and consensus. This hides the diversity of ideas, beliefs, and identities that constitute a community, the power asymmetries within, and the conflicts, struggles, and cooperation that result from these.

The lens of power exposes the hierarchies and conflicts that characterise communities rather than the commonalities many people expect within community life. Lukes (2005) extends a relational understanding of power and identifies its three faces: (1) where the powerful dictate the actions of others (decision-making); (2) the powerful set the rules on which terms issues are debated (non-decision-making); and (3) The powerless internalise the assumptions of the powerful about what is and is not possible (power over ideas). Disempowerment of communities can result from all these dimensions of power, with states and markets increasing social controls on the one hand and limiting possibilities for development on the other. Foucault sought to understand how power worked within communities by exploring the ways in which mechanisms of knowledge and power shape or discipline the subject, using increasingly sophisticated technologies of surveillance to create, classify, and control society (Gilchrist and Taylor 2016). For Foucault (1982), knowledge symbolised power. Having knowledge enables communities to challenge power structures and resist oppression. Thus, making knowledge accessible and generating awareness became a common thrust of much of the community development initiatives. In addition, several important theoretical contributions from feminism, post-structuralism, and post-colonialism help to understand the oppression experienced by marginalised communities.

Bourdieu's concept of habitus, described as the unconscious dispositions acquired through daily life (Davies 2011), has important implications to understand the inequalities within a community. Individuals acquire degrees of economic, social, and cultural capital depending on their background, education, wealth, networks, and other attributes and habitus structures. This privileges certain people over others, providing insights into power asymmetries within which communities. Bourdieu's work highlights how disadvantage is inbuilt into society's structures, and the patterns of inequalities and resulting tensions that exist within modern communities. This analysis of power sees an erosion of social capital and reflects Gramsci's view of civil society as the site where popular consent is engineered in societies, ensuring those with power retain privilege. However, Gramsci also saw civil society as an arena where hegemonic ideas could be contested, which provides the basis for radical conceptions of community development and participation.

One of the critical tensions in community organising and mobilisation concerns the issue of geography (that is, territorial affinities and resulting issues of distribution of resources, access and exclusion) versus the issue of oppression, discrimination, and systemic inequalities. The former are united by the pursuit of an apolitical vision of 'common good' while the latter demands resistance to societal hierarchies and assertion of marginalised identity.

Case study 3.1: Community participation: the case of the Landless Workers Movement

The Landless Workers Movement (Movimento dos Trabalhadores Rurais Sem Terra; MST) is a one of the largest social movements in Latin America, which seeks land reform in Brazil. The movement's aims are to redistribute land to rural workers for small-scale farming through large-scale land-occupation settlements (McCowan 2023). The ideology of the movement is shaped by Marxism and liberation theology and its core values are social justice, equality, cooperativism, environmental protection, sustainability, and (transforming the capitalist system). The movement was founded in 1984 at Cascavel in the southern Brazilian state of Paraná, although its origins go back to the peasant uprisings supported by radical Catholic Church groups during the 1960s. The movement has grown in scale, leading more than 2,500 land occupations with about 370,000 families, and has won nearly 18.75 million acres (7.5 million hectares) of land as a result of their direct action.

Brazil has huge inequalities in land distribution, with only 2 per cent of landowners having control of 50 per cent of all agricultural land (McCowan 2023). MST has used Article 184 of the Brazilian Constitution of 1988, which states that unused farmland should be expropriated and used for redistribution, to push for land distribution to peasant farmers. To pursue its aims, the movement's main tactic is land occupation but it also organises marches, demonstrations, and awareness-raising campaigns to bring the issue of agrarian reform to public attention.

This land occupation involves a group of landless people (between 500 and 3,000) going into a large estate and occupying the land. Given that it can take a long time for land rights to be granted by the government, temporary camps known as acampamentos are formed. The acampamentos are cooperatives that provide welfare services, including education, health, and food. If the claim for land rights is successful, an assentamento (settlement) is formed, whereby each family receives approximately 25 acres (10 hectares) of land. The movement originally hoped that land would be farmed collectively, though now families can choose between collective and individual farming, as long as there is some degree of collaboration.

MST is also active in education, with the creation of primary and adult education to address the high levels of illiteracy among the landless peasant communities. MST had more than 1,500 primary schools in its communities, which are financed and administered by municipal or state governments but follow the distinctive educational philosophy of the movement. These schools are based largely on the ideas of Paulo

Freire and follow the ethos of the MST movement, in terms of the commitment to the struggle for land reform and social justice in general.

Concept of participation and participatory development

The Landless Workers Movement (Case Study 3.1) and similar mobilisations elsewhere are based on the ideas of Paulo Friere (1970). For Friere, authentic participation directly addresses power and its distribution in society. Here the principal objective of the participation was not development – or poverty alleviation – but the transformation of the cultural, political, and economic structures which produce poverty and marginalisation (Leal 2007). Friere stressed the process of 'conscientisation', calling for raising awareness and organising those who are oppressed to assert their voice and progressively transform their environment through collective political action (Rahman 1993). As Friere argues, human beings are only free when they possess their own decision-making powers and are free of oppressive and dehumanising circumstances (Friere 1970). These ideas draw on the Marxist vision of self-emancipation of the oppressed classes. This included a view of development focused on the release of people's creativity rather than just economic growth. Paulo Friere offers one clear vision of participation.

Over the last two decades, grassroots organising and collective action by precarious communities has been growing. This has led to the emergence of grassroots organisations, which are involved in a variety of activities including income generation, campaigning, mutual aid or organising, to reforming institutions. The idea of community participation has been influenced by populist movements that champion the cause of ordinary people, with an emphasis on cooperative models of social and economic organisation (Worsley 1967).

However, the concept of participation is contested, and we see a very different vision of participation offered by agencies like the World Bank. Its definition of joining in involves the participation of ordinary people in existing development programmes to enhance their reach and acceptability; rather than addressing the structural factors that created the conditions that impede health in the first place (World Bank 1989). Here the idea of participation focuses more on ideas of 'empowerment' and self-reliance rather than political change (Leal 2007) needed to challenge the neoliberal system creating poverty. Calls for people to take control in such contexts also establish the need for people to be liberated from an interventionist state pursuing protectionist policies and take fuller charge of their lives by participating in development projects (Leal 2007).

This led to 'participatory development', characterised by a rapid growth of NGOs and foreign donor funded programmes promoting people's collective efforts taking form. Participatory development is increasingly being adopted as a more secure way of taking development to the people. Scholars highlight how this led to the co-option of more radical grassroots initiatives and marginalisation of more radical thinking and action towards empowerment and liberation (Kapilashrami and O'Brien 2012).

However, in the past two decades participation has been reframed as a rights issue, thus influencing many development agencies in their approach to participation. This view presents participation by the people in the institutions and systems which govern their lives as a basic human right and essential for realignment of political power in favour of disadvantaged groups and for social and economic development. Social participation is seen as a transformation of the traditional community development approach towards enhancing local people's capabilities to define and address their own needs and aspirations (WHO 2024a). Sen (1999) underscores the need of people to be actively involved in the process, with a focus being placed on the capability of the people.

The recently adopted landmark resolution on social participation (WHO 2024b) underscores the rights language, and emphasises community

Figure 3.2: Rights-based participatory development

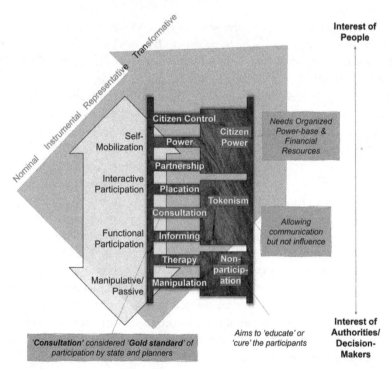

50

empowerment and inclusive participation in decision making processes that affect health.

Typologies of participation

Although any typology or model can be simplistic, it can be a useful way of understanding different forms of participation and in framing both the intention and approach behind them (Cornwall 2008).

Sherry Arnstein's (1969) ladder of participation is one of the most cited typologies that retains considerable contemporary relevance. Arnstein's model highlights the manipulations that can be inherent in participatory decision-making processes, providing a critique that centres on the extent to which power is devolved to participants. She describes a ladder of participation with linear steps from 'non-participation' aiming to 'educate' or 'cure' participants at the bottom; through 'tokenism' that allows communication but not influence; to increasing degrees of decision-making power as the ladder progresses. 'Consultation', considered the gold standard of engaging communities by planners and governments, may offer an ear to citizens' views but does not guarantee these will be heard, and continues to privilege powerholders. 'Citizen control' is the highest rung and occurs when participants in communities can be in full charge of the policy, programmes, and management that affect their lives. However, this requires an organised powerbase in the community and, ideally, financial resources.

Jules Pretty (1995) identifies 'bad' forms of participation, described as 'manipulative', as representing tokenistic inclusion with no real power, and 'passive' participation ensues the decisions that have already been made. The model then moves to functional participation, most often associated with efficiency arguments, where people participate to meet project objectives to reduce costs. The next stage is interactive participation, a learning process through which local groups take control over decisions. Finally, self-mobilisation is marked by people taking the initiative independently of external organisations, receiving assistance, but retaining control over these resources.

Both Arnstein's and Pretty's typologies describe a spectrum defined by a shift from control by authorities to control by the people or citizens. Yet, the endpoints are different. Pretty argues that participation may not challenge existing distributions of wealth and power. Indeed, local self-mobilisation may serve the interests of the state and international agencies within a neoliberal approach to development.

Sarah White (1996) offers some insights into the different interests at stake in various forms of participation. It prioritises the consideration of the interests (Who seeks participation and with what purpose? Who participates and why?) over the nature or extent of participation. Her main argument is that different types of participation serve different interests. To illustrate, 'nominal participation' legitimates the purpose of the people at the top, where participants may feel 'included' but the function of such participation is decorative, what she calls a 'display'. 'Instrumental participation' may deem engagement necessary, serving 'efficiency' interests and 'representative participation' ensures the 'sustainability' of projects for development planners. While White acknowledges that these forms of participation may give voices to the poor and marginalised, she asserts that 'transformative' participation leads to greater consciousness of what makes and keeps people poor and increased confidence in their ability to make a difference through empowerment (White 1996). Typologies such as these can be read as implicitly normative, suggesting a progression towards more 'genuine' or desired forms of participation that serve the interests of people (illustrated in Figure 3.2). Different purposes, equally, demand different forms of engagement by different kinds of participants. However, the normative goal of empowering publics remains unmet in many engagement processes. New thinking on participation needs to explain how it facilitates and subverts power relations between those participating.

Another conception of participatory process identifies two decisive ways in which the concept of participation can be viewed, especially in relation to development. Participation as a 'means' or participation as an 'end' (Cornwall 2008). The former implies engaging and mobilising communities primarily for the purpose of achieving a defined goal, for example, successful delivery of an intervention or informing local priorities and plans. Such view is critiqued for its failure to affect power relations between those at the grass roots and the decision makers (Parfitt 2004) and meet the empowerment goal of participation (Tufte and Mefalopulos 2009). Rather, communities are viewed as passive agents or tools that will help meet pre-defined goals and projects, while there is little or no relinquishing of power by the elite in the process (Rahnema 1992).

Participation as an end, on the other hand, regards the process as a core objective of engagement. It directs attention towards increasing the capacity of the participants to engage with political and other processes, while simultaneously addressing the contextual and structural barriers that impede meaningful participation. The latter demands breaking down existing barriers and constraints – political, social, and psychological – to people's participation (Oakley 1995), with the end goal of empowerment and power redistribution. Nikkhah and Redzuan, corroborating Asnarulkhadi (1996), defined participation as a process 'in which people are directly involved in shaping, deciding, and taking part in the development process from the bottom-up perspective' (2009, p 173). Participation thus becomes a 'process of achieving greater individual fulfilment, personal development, self-awareness, and some immediate satisfaction' (Nikkhah and Redzuan

2009, p 173). Collective action also builds capabilities to actively challenge the status quo or at least contemplate the system within which they reside.

The gap between the rhetoric and reality of participation

Referring to participatory development, few scholars regard participation as a tyrannical process, masking various aspects of power behind the rhetoric and practices of participation (Cooke 2003). Cooke and Kothari (2001, pp 7–8) identify three types of tyranny: decision-making tyranny manifested by the dominance of multinational agencies; group-level tyranny where practices of participation obscure inequalities and may contribute to the maintenance or increase in power differences; and methodological tyranny that reveals the dominance and overwhelming acceptance of participatory methods, despite limited space for meaningful participation. There are, however, acts and processes of participation (for example, sharing knowledge, negotiating day-to-day power relations, structural oppressions, and injustices within societies) that cannot be opposed through tyranny arguments (Cooke and Kothari 2001), although the authors argue that these acts and processes can conceal and reinforce oppressions and injustices within various practices of participation.

Notably, promoting the ideals of participation (often in building consensus through consultation with communities) can understate the political nature of policy processes. Frequently, issues that are most difficult to address – such as structural inequities of class, racism, and patriarchy – get ignored (Mohan and Stokke 2000; Mosse 2001). This raises the question of who participates (as well as who is excluded and who remain peripheral to participatory processes), and to what extent. Farrington and Bebbington (1993) propose a simple axis to assess forms of participation according to depth and breadth of engagement. A 'deep' participatory process engages participants in all stages of a given activity, from identification to decision-making. Such a process can remain 'narrow', however, if it only involves a handful of people, or particular interest groups. Equally, a 'wide' range of people might be involved, but if they are only informed or consulted their participation would remain 'shallow'. Such view is potentially useful to explore claims to participation that turn out to have involved only privileged and powerful (for example, rich, White, cis men) members of the 'community', and exclusion of other groups, such as poor women and children (Cornwall 2008). We examine these exclusions in Chapter 4.

Truism as it is, it is often far from obvious that most participatory processes do not and literally cannot involve 'everyone' and therefore may be exclusionary. In practice, who participates is determined by actions and methodologies that may be driven by implicit or explicit biases: distinctions between approaches that place greater emphasis on the participation of representatives – those who speak about and for a particular interest group – and those that seek more directly democratic forms of participation. In practice, these boundaries tend to be blurred. In most participatory consultation and planning work, pragmatism often dictates that the voices of some are to be taken to represent others, be they 'the poor' or 'the [undifferentiated] community'. This brings with it a host of further questions about representation and voice, aspects we explore in Chapter 5 on social movements, and Chapter 4 on inequities.

Although participation is seen as a noble ideal, nevertheless, in practice, participation often takes the form of enlisting people to secure their compliance in predetermined targets or implementing top-down agendas (White 1996; Cooke and Kothari 2001). Participation can be tokenistic in nature, where citizens seen as 'beneficiaries' are consulted on predetermined goals (Baines-Johnson and Bilici 2018). It has often been used to pay lip service 'for reasons of political expediency, and a real fear that grassroots organisations will generate popular empowerment beyond state control' (Brohman 1996).

Participation is now seen as a key component of social development programmes across the world, and is essential for strengthening the sense of citizenship among marginalised or excluded communities (Gaventa 2002; Mohan 2007). Structural problems including race, class, and caste have been core to community organising in different parts of the world. Assertion of particular marginalised identity allowed subordinate and marginalised social groups to organise and build social movements which went beyond class as the organising principle (Bernstein 2005). The lens of intersectionality (Crenshaw 2017) helped challenge universal conceptions of oppression based on singular identity and diversified formation and organising of feminist or identity-based movements. However, there is growing backlash of marginalised communities including migrants, people of different ethnicities and of different religious persuasions, and a rise of hostile identity politics and nationalist populism (Cox 2018; Singh 2021). The term gender backlash is now being increasingly used for actions that undermine progress towards gender equality (OHCHR n.d.) and focus primarily on demands of representation or determination. There is also a danger, as evidenced in several mainstream participatory development programmes, of prioritising the immediate or 'practical' needs of women 'without addressing the underlying aspects of gender subordination such as the unequal division or reproductive labour, restrictions on female mobility, domestic violence, women's lack of autonomy and so on' (Mayoux 1995, p 242).

There are several explanations for the rise of such inimical social and political forces in contemporary times. This includes undermining of the sense of identity of earlier times among the natives or erstwhile privileged groups, as well as extreme inequalities brought about by neoliberal globalisation. Others see it only as a political tactic of those who are keen to claim and hold on to power (Cox 2018). Community development practitioners and activists need to be cautious of such populism because it often employs a similar rhetoric of privilege and powerlessness and strategies like mobilising and organising that are used for facilitating the empowerment and participation of the marginalised in governance and development processes.

Community development and its theoretical underpinnings

Community development is linked with the development of democracy and civil society. At its heart, it must be driven by the grassroots and address needs identified by communities themselves. However, over the past 100 years, ideas of community development have evolved through the practices of community development initiatives, programmes, and policies in many parts of the world and embedded in colonial histories. Community organising entered the development discourse following the First World War when the colonial powers realised that they needed a framework under which the colonies could engage in development activity. For example, the British Government used the idea of community development as part of its colonial development projects to improve the living conditions of local populations through different forms of social development, such as health, education, and housing (Henderson and Vercseg 2010). In large parts of the colonised world, this was often accompanied by exploitation and extraction of natural and physical resources (Atampugre 1998; McCoy et al 2024).

A very different model emerged in the US, where Saul Alinsky mobilised communities in Chicago to improve their living conditions. Alinsky was based in inner-city Chicago in the 1930s. He brought together civic society groups, including unions and faith groups, to develop the Back of the Yards Neighbourhood Council. The council campaigned for several welfare programmes and facilities, including health prevention and child nutrition and advocated for improved pay and conditions for workers at the meatpacking company. Alinsky scaled up the community organising model by creating the Industrial Areas Foundation, which supported capacity building and training for community organisers in Chicago (Alinsky 1972).

With these two examples we witness the tensions that exist within much community development activity. On the one hand, community development can be led by the state to promote the participation of communities in welfare provision and improving their access to services. On the other hand, community development can be a grassroots social movement or initiative that involves communities identifying an issue of concern and then taking collective action to bring about social change (Henderson and Vercseg 2010). In the examples of community development discussed later in the chapter, there are examples of community development that fall into either category while there are others that bridge them.

Several key principles underpin community development ideas and practice. First, in terms of its normative scope and focus, community development demands tackling structural disadvantage, and the different forms of oppression prevalent in society, for instance, inequalities based on class, gender, and ethnicity (Stephney and Popple 2008). Tackling these unequal stratifications can lead to social change. However, community development emphasises the idea of change from below, or bottom-up development. This stresses that the community should be able to determine its own needs and how they should be met, thus owning the processes of planning and action. Critical to ensuring ownership and driving change from below is empowerment of communities, and their meaningful participation in processes of change.

Empowerment – an enabling process through which individuals and communities take control of their own lives and their environment (Rappaport 1984) –is both a conduit and an end goal of community development. Development workers strive to promote empowerment by equipping communities with the resources, opportunities, vocabulary, knowledge, and skills that enhance their capacity to effect change. While the endeavour is to maximise participation, with the aim being for everyone in the community to be actively involved in community processes and activities (Stephney and Popple 2008), in the next chapter we discuss the limits and possibilities for enabling such participation.

Finally, community development's goal of driving bottom-up change places utmost value on the 'local' knowledge, understandings, and capabilities. This inevitably shifts the focus to challenging imperialist and colonial ideas and extractive practices of development that have historically depleted local environments and disenfranchised communities (for example, First Nations people).

Different theoretical ideas and influences have shaped the emergence of community development as a field of practice. These influences were not mutually exclusive.

Marxist theories

There is a long tradition of Marxism as a philosophical influence on community development. Marxist ideas in community development, embodied in the works of Friere (1970) and Gramsci (1971), focus on the potential in communities for promoting solidarity through the collective struggle against capitalist oppression. This places community work within a wider struggle for policy and political change to counter oppression. It recognises civil society as the sphere for social change and is concerned with the re-democratisation of society. Radical Marxist models of community development have promoted strategic alliances between marginalised groups and the labour movement. They have turned to the discourse and critical dialogue models of Gramsci and Friere as a means of raising the consciousness of the powerless to challenge existing hegemonies and forms of systemic power. Gramsci saw change coming through education, cultural shifts, and the formation of social movements and highlighted the importance of 'political educators' as catalysts for change (Gilchrist and Taylor 2016). Critiques of Marxist community development highlight the limitations of local action in challenging the influence of powerful multinational companies and governmental agencies. It also overlooks the conflicting agendas between different oppressed groups, even to the point of some indigenous communities holding discriminatory views of new migrants, including refugees and asylum seekers. In addition, Marxist feminists have examined capital sources of women's oppression, an area that often remained neglected in Marxist mobilisation (Hartmann and Markusen 1980).

Feminist theory and praxis

Emerging from a critique of the androcentric focus and male bias inherent in labour movements and working-class struggles, women's movement and feminist practices have significantly enriched community development knowledge and practice, across the globe. As a result of the activism of working-class women from the 1970s, community development initiatives began incorporating feminist practices (Dominelli 2006).

Feminist community development interventions have strived to counter unequal gender power relations and raise critical consciousness of women's rights and how patriarchy and gendered norms, relations, and roles impact on access to and control over assets, health, and development at household, community, state levels, and globally. Such consciousness-raising within feminist community development draws on critical, collective, and participatory pedadgogies, and develops as women begin to situate and explain their everyday experiences within wider external structures of inequality and oppression (Robson and Spence 2011).

Examples of community activism and development that spin off from such feminists' anti-oppressive struggles are abound. Combahee River Collective, Southall Black Sisters and Brixton Black Women's Group in the UK, Autonomous women's movement, and the Dalit women's movement in India, among others. These engagements, and the ongoing interrogation of the unified meaning and experience of being a 'woman' (or the category of 'gender') have created a fertile ground for the birth of intersectionality theories (Crenshaw 2013; Davis 2015), particularly from the standpoint of the marginalised (Rege 1998; Simon-Kumar 2017; Anandhi and Kapadia

2017; Kapilashrami, Hill and Meer 2018). Tackling these intersectional inequalities through collective community action, while centring women, has the potential to accelerate the achievement of a more equal and just society.

Pluralist theories

The pluralist approach to community work theory and practice has been very prominent in recent times. Pluralist theories challenge the deterministic view adopted by the Marxist approach. Pluralists understand power within a democratic framework, where decisions are negotiated between different stakeholders (Gilchrist and Taylor 2016). The state is seen as having a mediating role in balancing the interests of different stakeholders. There is an important role for advocacy by civil society such as trade unions, political parties, religious groups, and social movements as centres of power and influence. Applied to community development, this approach focuses on supporting disadvantaged communities in making their voices heard and in becoming politically active, in order to advocate for their interests. Community development workers support communities to develop their confidence and skills, so they can organise collectively and advocate for their own interests. They also work with duty bearers to ensure they promote participation in their work with communities. This pluralist approach has been linked with the concept of communitarianism, which promotes social harmony through encouraging everyone to be active citizens and participate in building their communities (Stepney and Popple 2008). This influenced the emergence of 'third way' politics in the 1990s.

Critics of the pluralist approach have suggested it negates wider political analysis and ignores structural inequalities and power imbalances within society, suggesting its adoption as placatory and unlikely to lead to significant change (Popple 2015).

Post-modernist theories

Another theoretical influence on community development is the post-modernist or post-Enlightenment discourse. Enlightenment thinking has been a dominant discourse since the eighteenth century, as a basis for human reason and scientific objectivity (Edelstein 2010). However, it was seen as problematic with its focus on individualism, colonialism, capitalism, and top-down expertise (Ife 2013). Postmodernism is aligned with the theory of social constructionism, where ideas and meaning are contested by different stakeholders. Postmodernism questions the ideas of universality and challenges conventional bureaucratic wisdom that has led to top-down managerial practices and hierarchical control, which fits well with the principles of community development's horizontal ethos. However, community work practitioners have often mistrusted postmodernism as it challenges modernist frameworks such as human rights and social justice that are seen as fundamental to community development. However, rather than suggesting the concept of social justice is not of value, it proposes that such ideas are contested and open to different interpretations by different people in different circumstances, which are no longer static universal values but rather concepts people can come together to dialogue about and construct in a variety of ways. Esteva and Prakash (1998) argue that postmodernism has some very significant implications for community development. Its acceptance of diversity, and of messiness and contradiction, fits well with the reality of the experience of communities. It promotes the idea of 'relational reality' (Gergen 2000), in which relationships create reality and give meaning to the world. Moreover, it values the role of individual and community stories or narratives as catalysts for change within communities.

Social movement theory

Another key theory to influence community development is social movement theory, which is discussed further in Chapter 6. Social movements are described as 'claimed spaces', natural experiments in power, legitimation, and democracy. These movements have their roots in the oppositional movements that emerged in Europe in the early nineteenth century as a response to social upheaval and inhumane conditions wrought by the industrial revolution (Campfens 1997). Social movement theory explores the political opportunities for change, the ways in which resources are mobilised and how issues are framed (Gilchrist and Taylor 2016). It connects individuals' critical awareness of their situation with the need for collective action. Over the years, traditional social movements focused on class (based on the labour and trade union movement) have been joined by a new wave of social movements based on identity, that seek social and cultural transformation as well as political change. As we discuss in Chapters 5 and 9, the internet and social media have further transformed the potential and organisation of social movements. Castells (2012) describes how these new technologies have given birth to new forms of organisation and politics, supplementing and possibly supplanting the traditional political parties. These developments offer tremendous scope for community development work and opportunities for community development workers to widen their base and build solidarity.

In addition to these meta theories, several other concepts and theoretical ideas have shaped community development practice. Psychological and social learning theories offer insights into what motivates people within communities, how knowledge is processed and how people act. Theorists in this tradition have argued that knowledge is derived from experience and validated in practice (Campfens 1997), suggesting a dialectical cycle in which existing theory is influenced by lessons from practice, which in turn are applied to the process of action. Group development and dynamics (Tuckman 1965) and other human behaviour theories, including Maslow's hierarchy of needs, have also informed effective processes of group formation, and individual motivation for collective action affecting social change. Most notably, ideas of mutual aid, human solidarity, and communitarianism advanced by social anarchists like Proudhon (1979) and Kropotkin (1989) are other critical influences. Rejecting all forms of authority, especially that of the state, these writings aspired to create alternative, self-governing communities. The communitarian tradition has sustained societies throughout history, as seen in clans, medieval guilds, and agricultural communities. These ideas resurged to prominence with the emergence of self-help groups and mutual support networks in the nineteenth and twentieth centuries, fundamentally shaping political thinking with the advent of third way political philosophy that is neither market- nor state-led. There is a clear role for community development in supporting the development of self-help and mutual aid through bringing people with a shared interests together and creating the structures for these networks to flourish.

Globalisation and neoliberal economics had considerable impact upon communities in terms of uncertainty, greater fragmentation, and less solidarity. This has provided a new impetus for community development through the emergence of new social movements to challenge the impact of neoliberalism and meet the gap in provision created by neoliberalism. The internet is allowing people to connect both locally and globally, that have resulted in rapid spread and growth of movements opposed to discrimination, such as Black Lives Matter, #MeToo, and the disability movement. These counter movements have attempted to recreate and connect with notions of community. According to Cohen and Rai (2000), global social movements represent a post-national phase with political action becoming more unconventional, open, direct, participatory, and focused. These movements link local and global struggles that are addressing key issues including women's movements, peace movements, labour movements, and environmental movements. Some movements have extensive international networks, whereas others are smaller in scale. The anti-globalisation movement has made connections between different issues, including the environmental crisis, poverty, race, and gender discrimination. However, there remain significant barriers in connecting struggles across national boundaries, and economic divides, limiting the potential for social and political change. These include state controls and surveillance, resources, inequities in access to technological revolution, and more siloed nature of activism and advocacy that we further discuss in Chapter 5.

The practice of community development in an international context

Community development practices have evolved under various influences across different parts of the world. While a comprehensive historical overview is outside the scope of this book, we examine some of these developments below, charting a brief history of community development today.

Western Europe and North America

The Western experience of community development largely came from the desire to rebuild a war-ravaged Europe and witnessed its incorporation into state interventions. This began with the work of the settlements at the beginning of the twentieth century and after the Second World War it involved setting up community centres in new council estates to improve social connections and tackle social issues, such as poor housing. In the 1960s, a more radical community development initiative known as the National Community Development Project was established to tackle poverty and urban deprivation (Henderson and Vercseg 2010). Project teams investigated causes of social problems in areas of deprivation and developed community work responses to address these issues. Community development continued in the 1980s and 90s that supported the development of a mixed economy of welfare under the Conservatives and as a way of creating harmony and social cohesion during the New Labour Government. The Conservative governments post-2010 adopted community development as part of a strategy of shrinking the state and shifting responsibility for welfare provision on to communities.

A similar trend was witnessed in other parts of Europe, with community development incorporated within both social work and adult education professions in France, within urban renewal programmes in the Netherlands and Belgium and welfare provision in Ireland. A Europe-wide community development collaboration was established in the 1990s, which also drew in cooperative movements in Italy and adult education initiatives in Scandinavia.

Community development in the US grounded in the anti-war and civil rights movement in the 1960s and emerged as part of the government's war on poverty. Community organising developed to support citizen participation in planning and decision-making in neighbourhoods, empowering communities to challenge racial discrimination and combat poverty. Neighbourhood organisations set up and developed initiatives like community enterprise and community banking.

Since the 1990s there has been a growing emphasis on community capacity building and an asset-based approach to community development (Kretzmann and McKnight 1993).

In the Central and Eastern Region, a long tradition of community development exists as evidenced in practices of self-help groups, associations, and workers' movements. Under socialist regimes from 1945–1989, community development explicitly targeted community education and cultural houses and settlement activities[1] in places like Hungary and Romania, which were meeting places for use by local communities. These democratic spaces became a conduit of political development of communities and activism. The intellectual also had a strong role to play and involved galvanising people into social action in several countries including Hungary, Poland, and the Czech Republic. In Hungary, for example, intellectuals helped create the Hungarian public education and community development movement. The collapse of communism in the late 1980s saw the re-emergence of community development.

Community development experiences in the (post)colonial world

Albeit less visible or cited in mainstream scholarship on community development, freedom struggles and nation building in post-colonial states in the Global South have offered critical insights into the development of CD. Work of the Brazilian adult educationalist, Paulo Friere, for instance, has greatly influenced community development practice globally. This helped stimulate a rapid growth in grassroots organisations in Latin America (that were distinctly anti-state), and development assistance for impoverished people, based on self-help principles and underpinned by a radical discourse.

Similarly, community development informed approaches have been used for a range of development purposes including poverty alleviation, literacy, family planning, nutrition, primary healthcare, and income-generating projects. These are aimed at both the rural and urban poor sometimes with specific focus on special groups like women or landless peasants (Campfens 1997). While community development across the Global South often approached along similar lines, the diversity of communities and complexity of development in these countries, many of whom were colonised till recently, is illustrated with the case of India.

Case study 3.2: Community development practices: the case of India

In India, community development evolved primarily as a response and challenge to colonial rule. Even though influenced by enlightenment ideas, they reflected indigenous concerns and locally embedded traditions and aimed to strengthen a national identity. After independence, 'community development' was appropriated as a formal strategy of nation building with the introduction of the Community Development Block as the lowest unit of rural development. However, rights-based approaches to community development which had been incorporated into government practice are increasingly under strict scrutiny. The current situation in India emphasises the contextual and deeply political nature of community development and participatory practice.

The many influences on community development

India is a nation today, but 75 years ago it was a dominion of the British Empire with a deeply feudal society. Its shadow exists to this day. Society continues to be organised by caste and tribal identities and segregated along strict gender and patriarchal divisions. One of the core challenges in a newly independent state was to forge a common 'national' identity. Over the years this national identity in India has become conflated with a 'Hindu' identity, alienating Muslims. This is a legacy of partition into secular India and Islamic Pakistan. There have been multiple waves of 'othering' based on place of origin, birthplace, religion, language spoken both at the national level and in states (provinces). The search for a common Indian 'identity' continues to influence contemporary politics and ongoing contestations around who is a citizen.

A range of social and political influences have shaped the wider context in which identity formation occurred. For instance, the strong wave of social reform influenced by the enlightenment ideas that accompanied the advent of Europeans was visible in resisting oppressive practices of sati and so on. Later a counter-reform movement began, and efforts to change traditional practices were seen as interference with religion. This tension between 'secular' social reform and traditional religious customs and beliefs has increased in recent years. The strain has increased as religious philanthropy and development activities of faith-based organisations widened in scope and influence on political organisations, changing the very character of development.

Another influence was a strong indigenous vision of community development, led by two key architects Rabindranath Tagore, the poet and Nobel Laureate, and Mahatma Gandhi, taking form. The Swadeshi Movement announced in 1905 was a political call for a boycott of British produced goods that also led to a strengthening of the Indian cottage industry. Both Gandhi and Tagore took these ideas forward in their own ways. Tagore started small experiments in rural reconstruction introducing voluntarism and cooperative actions, revival of cottage industries, as well as sanitation and hygiene initiatives (Chattopadhyay 2018). Gandhi's focus was on Sarvodaya (the welfare of all) and Gram Swarajya (village self-governance). He established spaces where people lived together and practiced self-sufficiency. These ideas continue to influence the work of NGOs throughout the country and inspired the 'Panchayati Raj' system of local governance that exists today.

Post independence, several political movements and localised resistance were led by communists focusing on land tenure systems and poverty like the Tebhaga or Naxalbari movement in Bengal or the Telangana Movement in erstwhile Andhra Pradesh. The JP movement in the 1970s in Bihar had its roots in Gandhian philosophy, but inspired a whole generation of youth activists who went on to lead political parties and NGOs. These struggles continue to inspire local mobilisations.

Community development in independent India

After independence the government introduced various programmes and schemes aimed at rural development, and tackling poverty, inequality, and deprivation. Often these had clear political underpinnings. The Gandhian tradition continued and was initially a close ally of the government. In 1975 Indira Gandhi clamped 'Emergency' and for a period of 18 months all civil and political rights were suspended. This became an important marker of state-civil society relationships. Laws introduced to regulate the receipt of foreign grants by independent organisations have become an important instrument of state control over civil society action in more recent years.

After the Emergency there has been a steady growth of voluntary action (and processes of reclaiming political spaces) throughout the country. Many were initiated by urban middle-class professionals. This was a new phase of autonomous nation building, influenced by but distinct from earlier historical political trends. Around this time the term 'NGO' emerged in the international development arena and soon was applied to these organisations in India. The 'development sector' grew through the 90s and by the turn of the millennium had become firmly established in the field of community development. This period also witnessed the entry of several International NGOS (INGOs) registering country offices and regarded as leading national organisations. The political, financial, and symbolic power wielded by these large INGOs supported by international donors and the resulting marginalisation of smaller indigenous organisations has been seen as a new form of colonisation (Cohen Kupcu and Khanna 2009).

A counter trend was the emergence of rights-based struggles within the 'development' arena. From the 80s onwards several issue-based people's movements, challenging the impact of development projects, started in different parts of the country. Notable among them were the Narmada Bachao Andolan (NBA), a movement of tribal communities against dam-related displacement, the Chipko movement against deforestation of the Himalayas, the anti-nuclear movement, the fisher people's movements, anti-mining movements, and the movement for compensation and healthcare by communities affected the Bhopal gas leak, one of the biggest industrial disasters globally. While being rooted in communities, they are seen as anti-establishment.

Two social identity-based movements that supported these struggles are the women's movement and the caste-based movements. These have contributed significantly to rights-based development and advocacy. Social mobilisation and welfare activities by Christian church-based organisations, influenced by liberation theology from Latin America, contributed to the strengthening of the dalit movement. Many of the constituents of the women's and dalit movement have assumed a civil society organisation character.

While civil society initiatives have addressed development issues among all communities, the Muslim community remained largely ignored. Since the time of partition, being Muslim is considered a political identity rather than a social identity. This meant unlike for the rural, the poor, or tribal or dalit population, which have received specific attention by facilitating individuals or agencies, the Muslim community even though poor and socially marginalised has remained ignored (Rahman 2018).

Contemporary challenges

Working with rural communities in India is often like working with multiple worlds at the same time. Signs of a modern, globalised world and traditions and customs coexist. Past feudal traditions are now transformed to client-patron relationships fostering corruption as well silence and complicity. Alongside an increasing polarisation of communities with the rise of the religious right-wing, violent assertions of the Hindu religious and political identity have affected the largely 'secular' civil society organisations as well.

Adapting and evolving and in the face of many challenges, the indigenous civil society has also assumed a multi-dimensional character. The same development actors can simultaneously or at different times be found in different spaces including in social movements, in indigenous NGOs, in international organisations, and as quasi-governmental spaces. Often this is seen as co-optation and at other times subversion. In difficult times, this flexibility is a survival strategy.

The relationship between the state and civil society has been collaborative as well as antagonistic. Economic liberalisation and associated privatisation created new dynamics in this relationship. With the state withdrawing from some of its public welfare functions, the NGO gained legitimacy in provision of services. Human rights defenders are seen as confrontational and even as 'anti-nationals', while organising and action by poor and marginalised communities (for example, landless farmers) to claim rights are construed as anti-state activities.

Conclusion

This chapter has discussed 'community development' to frame our understanding of this approach to practice that we explore in the rest of the book. The chapter illustrates the contested nature of both concepts of 'community' and 'community development'. While cognisant of the different approaches to engaging communities for development, we identify key principles that can be applied to the field of public health and health rights. This includes the crucial importance of power when understanding the nature of community and how communities can take action to address these power imbalances. The discussion in this chapter highlights how this approach can be applied within a public health context for transformative social change but also emphasises the limits too, given the wider structural issues that lead to entrenched oppression and disadvantage for marginalised populations.

The case study from India illustrates the huge potential, but also diverse influences, tensions, and evolving practices of community development. It indicates the layers of communitarian practices and organising that existed within society; some exclusionary and discriminatory, while others cooperative and transformative. We call for the need to develop more contextualised understandings that are mindful and respectful of these complex realities of post-colonial contexts and the marginalised communities that developed through political and social struggles.

The issue of power and empowerment is crucial to this analysis and the different typologies highlight how these complexities play out in practice. What clearly emerges is a gap between the rhetoric and reality of participation in several ways. The discussion raises the need to carefully assess the objectives of participatory process, and to distinguish rights-based and activism-oriented ideas of participation from the technical forms promoted by many development agencies. In the remaining sections, we explore the role of participation in tackling health inequalities and advancing health rights; for which awareness of these complexities is vital.

PART II

Pathways to health justice: community organising, collective action, and accountability

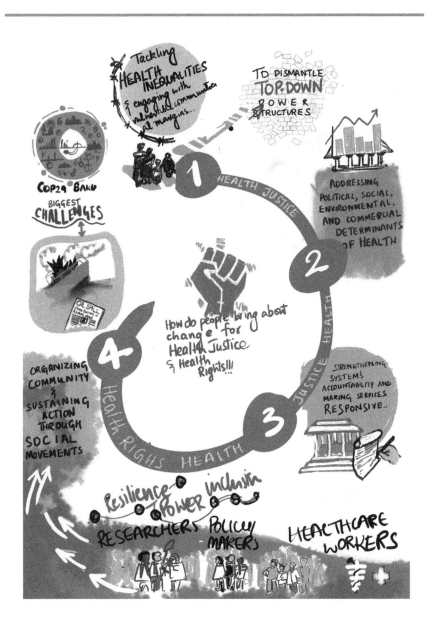

4

Engaging communities at the margins to reduce health inequalities

Health inequities: who are left behind? Who loses?

On average and in optimal conditions, a girl born in Hong Kong can expect to live 32 years longer than a girl born in Chad or Central African Republic. Differences across countries, in particularly the Global North and South, reveal historic injustices on a global scale; namely imperial pursuits, slavery and extractive development, and structural adjustments within neoliberal economic globalisation that weakened public institutions in countries. However, in the current global architecture, not all differences in health can be explained by power imbalances across nations. Inequalities within national borders tell another story.

In Scotland's most populous city, Glasgow, the train route from northwest (Jordanhill) to southeast (Bridgton) of Glasgow is telling. As per Figure 4.1, every station in this route signals a drop in life expectancy by two years for men and 1.2 years for women, totalling a 14- and 9-year difference in life chances of survival for men and women in the same city (McCartney 2011). Referred to as the Glasgow Effect, the phenomenon is attributed to a number of factors that cannot be simply linked to individual 'behaviours' or 'lifestyles'. These distal determinants include: a high prevalence of premature and low birthweight births, a high level of derelict land contaminated by toxins, more deindustrialisation than in comparable cities, higher levels of poverty, poor social housing, religious sectarianism, lack of social mobility, adverse childhood experiences, and social alienation (Ali 2012).

Another illustrative case of such inequalities is maternal health. As per 2018 estimates, maternal mortality rate (MMR), that is, maternal deaths per 100,000 live births ranged from two in Norway to 1,150 in South Sudan. So, the likelihood of a woman dying in childbirth in South Sudan is 575 times higher than a woman in Norway; 94 per cent of all maternal deaths occur in lower middle-income countries that are characterised by weak and poorly resourced health systems, poverty, and poor nutrition levels of mothers. Not all maternal deaths can be explained by a country's GDP or economic status. For instance, the United States with MMR of 17.4 ranks

Figure 4.1: Spatial map of health inequalities

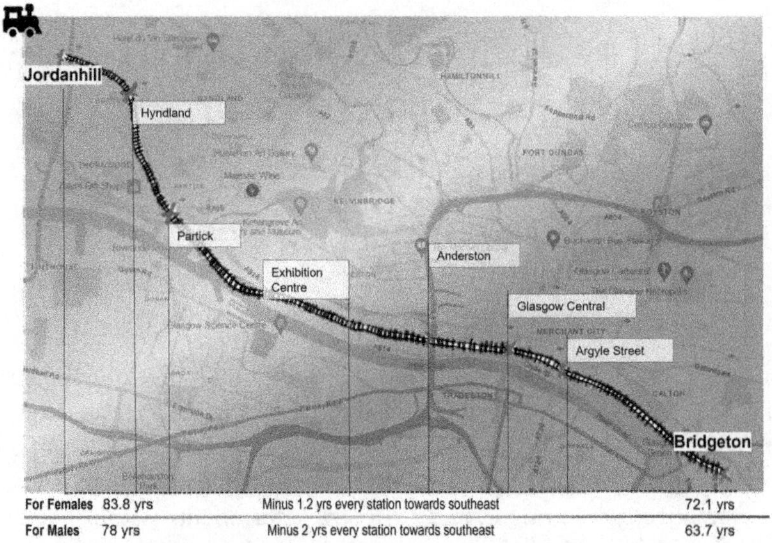
Jordanhill
Hyndland
Partick
Exhibition Centre
Anderston
Glasgow Central
Argyle Street
Bridgeton
For Females 83.8 yrs
Minus 1.2 yrs every station towards southeast
72.1 yrs
For Males 78 yrs
Minus 2 yrs every station towards southeast
63.7 yrs

Source: The Glasgow Effect – Spatial Map of Drop in Life Expectancy, modification of the original illustration by McCartney 2011

55th in the world, and last among similarly wealthy countries. These deaths result from a combination of gender-blind, coercive policies, state of health systems including extent of privatisation that drives unethical practices (for example, unnecessary treatments and over-medicalisation) and inequities in access, and low prioritisation of health.

Within country differences in maternal health tell another story. Maternal deaths are rare in the UK, fewer than 1 death in 10,000 pregnancies. However, some groups, especially women from minority ethnicities, bear a higher risk and disproportionate burden of pre-term birth, stillbirth, neonatal death, or a baby born with low birth weight (MBRRACE-UK 2022). In comparison to White British women, Black women are five times and Asian women two times more likely to die because of complications in their pregnancy (MBRRACE-UK 2022) and have significantly increased odds (83 per cent higher among black African women as compared to white European women) of severe maternal morbidity or long-term pregnancy-related complications (Lindquist et al 2013; Nair et al 2014). Confidential enquiry reveals multiple structural biases in UK maternity care, manifested in the form of micro-aggressions, and lack of clinically, socially, and culturally nuanced care received (Knight et al 2022).

These 'systematic differences in the health of people occupying unequal positions in society' are referred to as health inequalities (Graham 2009). These differences are not random or by chance, and result from a combination of historical and contemporary processes (such as colonialism, neoliberal economic globalisation, austerity 'reforms', and extractive development) that remain outside individual control. These macro forces stratify society into unequal positions that determine unequal access to healthcare and other determinants of health (such as nutrition, education, drinking water, sanitation) and result in unfair and preventable differences in health. As Michael Marmot argues, 'to understand why health is distributed the way it is, you have to understand society' (Marmot 2015, p 7).

The social environment we live in is widely recognised as shaping patterns of health and illness within and across populations. Understanding the factors, processes, and institutions through which these patterns are shaped and states of (ill)health produced therefore becomes necessary for developing appropriate policy and systems responses for well-being. However, conventional understandings of what these unequal positions are and what determines these differences are based on and tend to privilege single axis of vulnerability or an individual's social location (Kapilashrami 2022). For example, in the UK, scholarship and policy on health inequalities focuses predominantly on area-based deprivation, which is concerned with distribution of health by social class or socio-economic position and place of residence (Kapilashrami et al 2016; Kapilashrami and Marsden 2018). In the US, race and ethnicity is prominent in inequalities scholarship, while in large parts of the post-colonial world, the locus of enquiry is based on geography (rural–urban), caste (in the case of South Asia), indigeneity (First nations), gender, and/or, more recently, sexual identity, and disability-based disparities (Baru et al 2010).

We also know that people experience marginalisation and structural disadvantage along multiple dimensions/axes that are constantly shifting and re-configuring. For instance, conflict, disasters, and state policies introduced to tackle some of the challenges may produce or increase vulnerabilities of specific communities. Yet, the tendency to treat these vulnerabilities as static, predetermined, and operating in silos is commonplace in scholarly and policy debates. It is argued that privileging of one aspect of social location or axis of vulnerability over others undermines other dimensions of marginality as well as their interactions, leading to partial understanding of the distribution of ill-health and its determination in society (Kapilashrami 2022). Intersectionality has emerged as an alternative paradigm to conceptualise and address these multiple and interacting social positions and their effects (Crenshaw 1989). As discussed in the first chapter, a particular strength of this framework is to link the individual level experiences of marginality and disadvantage with the institutions, systems and structural processes that create these (Kapilashrami and Hankivsky 2018).

Different kinds of marginalisations exist in society today that produce inequities – people may experience structural disadvantage on the basis of living in remote areas, belonging to historically oppressed or stigmatised groups, those who are seen as 'interlopers' – immigrants, those who are discriminated or critiminalised for their sexuality, and various intersections between them. Further, groups who experience negative stereotyping and, consequently, exclusion including LGBT+ (Khanday and Akram 2012; Sekoni, Jolly, and Gale 2022). People who are part of marginalised population groups, whether based on 'race' or ethnicity, religion, language, migrant status, sexual orientation, or gender identity, have consistently been shown to exhibit poor physical and mental health outcomes on a range of measures (Marmot et al 2008; Wilkinson and Pickett 2010; Hughto, Reisner, and Pachankis 2015; González-Agüero et al 2018; Akintunde, Oladipo, and Oyaromade 2019).

A range of explanations are put forward for what determines poor health and the disproportionate (or excess) burden of disease among marginalised groups. To understand these, we go back to the stratifications and the social determinants of health. We know that multiple structural, contextual, and individual factors determine social disadvantage and affect health experience. These factors and pathways of determination of poor health have been captured in several frameworks that illustrate the complex ways in which social-political-economic and environmental factors interact to produce differences in health and well-being; as depicted in the conceptual framework by Solar and Irwin (2010) for action on the social determinants of health (Figure 4.2).

Structural factors impeding access to healthcare include poverty, unemployment, and poor housing, limited geographic and financial access to healthcare, and cultural factors include culturally inappropriate services, poor health literacy, and language barriers (Burhansstipanov, Dixon, and Roubideaux 2001; English et al 2006; Riggs et al 2012). Certain groups face multiple structural and cultural barriers, such as minority ethnic communities and people experiencing homelessness. Additionally, they often have higher risk factors for diseases, lack of awareness of the existing health resources, and are deemed 'hard to reach' (either physically or in terms of social discrimination), further limiting their access to healthcare (Balcazar et al 2009; Fawcett et al 2013). We saw these multiple disadvantages experienced by vulnerable groups during the COVID-19 pandemic. The 'hard to reach' reference however masks the systematic exclusion or oppression and chronic poverty resulting from failed promises of development, and oppression faced by certain populations (for example, in terms of racial and ethnic inequalities) that generates deep distrust in state and public facilities. These communities experience inequality in health outcomes and service access due to their marginalised social location (based on ethnic, religious or other minority identity) or structural conditions (unemployment, joblessness, homelessness). These groups can experience more severe exclusion in some countries compared to others depending on factors such as political power, historical oppression, and stereotyping.

Figure 4.2: CSDH framework for social determinants of health

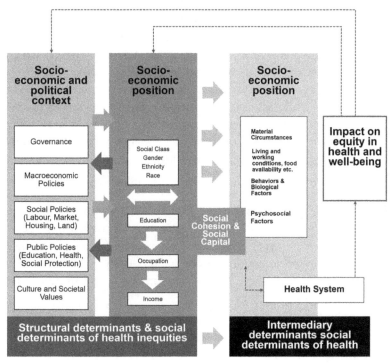

Source: Adaptation of final form of CSDH Framework for Social Determinants of Health by Solar and Irwin (2010)

Community engagement and collaborative priority setting are important for research to have a genuinely positive impact on the health of marginalised populations (Bonevski et al 2014). Health research can often be extractive and fail to consider the health agendas and priorities of the people who are being researched. Poorer, often stigmatised groups are often not included in healthcare planning, resulting in growing unmet needs in this population group. India's maternal health programme (Case Study 4.1) provides an interesting example of a globally successful 'model', where the experiences of the most marginalised communities were ignored and never separately considered during the planning, implementing, and monitoring stages (Das 2017).

Case study 4.1: Inequities in India's maternal health programme

India launched an ambitious maternal health programming called the Janani Suraksha Yojana (JSY) or Maternal Safety Scheme in 2005. This scheme which promoted universal Institutional Delivery was aimed at improving both maternal and newborn survival and contribute to India's efforts towards meeting MDGs 4 and 5. The rates of Institutional Delivery or hospital-based childbirth increased steeply, but the anticipated decline in maternal mortality and infant mortality among the most vulnerable did not happen (Lim et al 2010). Several studies highlighted that quality of services or referral had not improved (Chaturvedi et al 2014), especially for those living at the margins like urban slum-dwellers (Vikram, Sharma, and Kannan 2013), and other minority communities (Nasir 2014). An in-depth study among forest dwelling tribal population showed that the health system was completely ignorant of the health belief systems and healthcare practices of the community and compelled them to take unfamiliar measures (Contractor and Das 2015). All this happened even though community-based mobilisation was one of the key strategies adopted within the programme.

Such healthcare planning, and research that informs it, risks widening inequities by not prioritising those most in need (or with complex health needs) and is itself a form of marginalisation. These inequities are maintained by marginalised populations not exercising their health rights or not knowing who to complain to and how, often due to an absence of awareness-raising by state and non-state sectors.

Barriers to meaningful engagement of communities on the margins

Despite the inclusion of community engagement strategies and the obvious benefits of community development and participation, there are a number of problems and barriers to effective participation of communities, especially those 'on the margins'.

Healthcare programming is increasingly being driven by an 'evidence-based' paradigm. In most cases evidence-based paradigm requires a quantitative understanding of community-based realities and followed by a quantitatively driven monitoring and evaluation process. An example of this was the MDG process for stimulating international development within which there were eight goals and several numerical targets and indicators. Healthcare programming was implied in multiple goals like those related to child survival, maternal health, HIV/AIDS, TB, and malaria. The SDG process makes the goal and target setting even more elaborate with 18 goals and over one hundred targets and indicators. The data systems that are set up to serve these targets and indicators generate summaries, and at best provide some levels of disaggregation, often limited to rural-urban, and province-based differences. These data systems miss the realities of the communities at the margins, their experiences, and their realities.

There has been a proliferation of initiatives to engage communities at multiple levels, for example, in direct delivery of services, planning, and policy levels. Evidence suggests that service providers do not effectively engage disadvantaged communities in programmes designed to improve their health and instead engage with majority (white, high-income) populations on their needs instead (Sheikh 2006; Cochran et al 2008). Wallerstein (2006) reported that traditional health promotion programmes are often not designed in a culturally sensitive way, or fail to consider the disempowering conditions faced by disadvantaged populations that prevent them from engaging in the first place.

The dominant social participation approach is ineffective in reaching marginalised populations. Studies have shown that the majority of the health programmes use 'top-down' community engagement approaches, (often invoked in donor-driven health promotion programmes and limited to one-off consultations with communities on pre-designed programmes), as opposed to 'bottom-up' participatory approaches driven by communities. These approaches particularly disadvantage communities on the margins as they have been designed based on the needs of majority populations. This was discussed in Chapter 2, which presented evidence that participation in most interventions is limited to gathering evidence or 'Data' and engaging communities in 'Dialogue', with little evidence of involvement in the 'Decision' or 'Evaluation' stage where communities can be involved in reviewing and re-setting priorities (Arthur, Saha, and Kapilashrami 2023).

A second barrier for meaningful participation is the overwhelming focus on raising awareness of risk behaviours and lifestyles of individuals. Characteristic of most public health programmes engaging communities, such focus fails to engage in a redistribution of political power, economic wealth, and social recognition in order to create contexts that enable the poor health of marginalised groups to be addressed. However, rather than calling on power holders to affect such redistribution, public health programmes usually operate within the parameters of unequal power between service providers and communities (Campbell 2020). Moreover, implementing participation has highlighted the inadequacy of the health (and social) care system in supporting inclusive participation processes.

Meaningful implementation of community participation requires dedicated and sensitised staff with expertise in community development or community organising who have the time to work with communities to identify their needs and decide on a programme of collective action to address these needs. Without this, the process risks being tokenistic. The attitudes and behaviours of health professionals especially in relation to disadvantaged and stigmatised populations are critical barriers to community participation. In many contexts, health professionals are unwilling to relinquish their power, derived from their biomedical training and hierarchical systems in which they operate, to enable communities to shape the agenda. Some health professionals view community participation as an intervention to be managed and controlled by them within the health agency rather than as a process of engaging communities to set their own priorities and take action on the wider social determinants of health (Rifkin 2009).

We therefore argue that even well-intentioned, empowerment-focused initiatives that engage communities are unable to reach those that are hardest hit being multiply disadvantaged and may, in fact, even exacerbate the marginalisation they experience. Previously, we acknowledge how communities are a reflection of the wider power imbalance in societies and mirror the processes of social exclusion. Those 'left behind' include those experiencing chronic precarity and transience, historical marginalisation, including dispossession of their land and systemic discrimination (including racial and ethnic minorities, displaced populations, refugees, Roma and rural poor migrants, scavenging communities among others). These factors and experiences limit their reach and utilisation of healthcare and other entitlements. For instance, indigenous populations such as Maasai in Tanzania who report poorer maternal and child health outcomes (Lawson et al 2014) and lowest uptake of reproductive information and contraceptives (Carroll and Kapilashrami 2020). Given their historic marginalisation, these populations have limited trust in public health systems, and are most disconnected from and missed by programmes, services, and planning efforts (Lawson et al 2014).

Promising practices centering people's voices

With our understanding of both the benefits of and limits to participation, we explore some promising practices and their key ingredients of engaging marginalised communities that we draw on from different parts of the world.

The first example deals with addressing the barrier of donor-driven top-down programmes through mobilising and involving marginalised populations in the delivery of primary healthcare. This involves consulting with local communities on priorities for taking action on health and the design of healthcare interventions and then involving these communities at all stages of implementation of healthcare delivery. These pilots can then be evaluated and scaled up to transform national healthcare implementation and ensure more accessible services for communities on the margins.

Case study 4.2: The Navrongo Health Research Centre

The Navrongo Health Research Centre is located in the Kassena-Nankana East District of northern Ghana close to the border with Burkina Faso. In 1994, a community-based research project was initiated to develop, test, and evaluate approaches to rural health service delivery using a combination of strategies (http://www.ghana-chps.org/navrongo.htm).

Figure 4.3: Addressing barriers to effective engagement of communities at margin

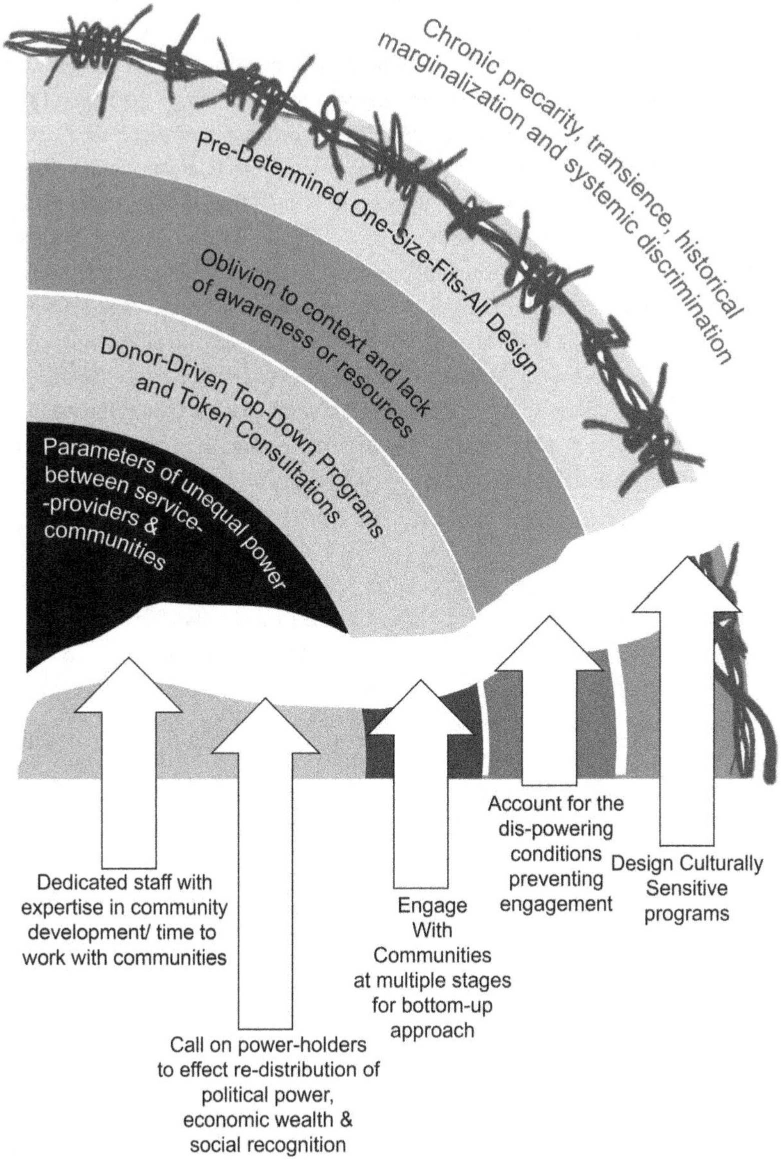

Chronic precarity, transience, historical marginalization and systemic discrimination

Pre-Determined One-Size-Fits-All Design

Oblivion to context and lack of awareness or resources

Donor-Driven Top-Down Programs and Token Consultations

Parameters of unequal power between service- -providers & communities

Dedicated staff with expertise in community development/ time to work with communities

Call on power-holders to effect re-distribution of political power, economic wealth & social recognition

Engage With Communities at multiple stages for bottom-up approach

Account for the dis-powering conditions preventing engagement

Design Culturally Sensitive programs

With the support and approval of the Ministry of Health, the Centre embarked on a series of consultations with the chiefs and residents of the district, who contributed to the design of the project, known as the Navrongo Experiment. The initiative made community leaders local consultants to the project and involved them at all stages of implementation. The process of consulting local authorities, opinion leaders, and household heads about any new activity in the community, including research, follows a long-established protocol that has become a model for public health interventions in Ghana. This approach has been incorporated into a policy known as the Ghana Community-Based Health Planning and Services Initiative, which has been adopted by several districts within the country. Unique features of the Navrongo model include community entry, a process of going into the community to meet with community leaders before initiating a research activity, and community 'durbars'. Durbars involve a gathering of chiefs, elders, opinion leaders, and community members, along with researchers, to deliberate on a proposed research agenda and to consolidate and communicate community views and concerns. Durbars have been used to mobilise the community for discussions about proposed projects, which demonstrates how cultural institutions can be utilised for mobilising communities and promoting the exchange of ideas. The Navrongo model allowed the community to participate in the process of understanding their health-related problems and at the same time develop appropriate solution. Subsequently the Ghana Community-based Health Planning and Services (CHPS) Initiative scales up innovations from this pilot study into a programme of national community healthcare reform (Nyonator et al 2005).

One of the important barriers faced by marginalised communities is a lack of knowledge about their health rights and entitlements. That is critical for effectively navigating health services and obtaining appropriate healthcare. Health rights specify which healthcare–related services and medical treatments people are entitled to receive, the choices they can make regarding what might be more appropriate for them, and how they can contest administrative decisions. Yet many people are unaware of or find it difficult to access information related to these, understand, and realise their health rights (Edgman–Levitan and Cleary 1996). This becomes an even greater challenge when information is inaccessible or culturally inappropriate and insensitive to specific needs. These barriers and strategies to address them are described in Figure 4.3.

Case study 4.3: Health information rights

A model drawing on a culture-centred approach was used to develop and present health rights information materials for a disadvantaged cultural minority – the Ethiopian immigrant community in Israel (Guttman, Gesser-Edelsburg, and Aycheh 2013). The model is based on the supposition that the design of health rights information materials should address both concerns and barriers identified by members of the cultural community and illustrate specific means to address them. At the time this model was implemented there were over 130,000 Ethiopians in Israel. They faced many hardships in their immigration process to Israel, including long stays at refugee camps, physical attacks, and even death of their family members. The public systems of Israel were very unfamiliar. Many didn't know Hebrew. They felt ignored, misunderstood, and discriminated against by healthcare providers. To build their confidence and self-esteem, stories of community members' actual experiences were collected. These then served as the basis for developing several types of narratives and presented in the form of video clips, a photo-novella, and an illustrated booklet. These were then presented among the Ethiopian immigrants to familiarise them with their health rights. Findings indicated participants felt the materials developed using this approach were informative and represented their concerns and cultural barriers to realising these rights from their perspective and would help motivate them to realise their health rights.

People need to have the capacities to understand and manage the system as well and the example of the Ethiopian immigrants provides how this can be made possible. This type of knowledge is referred to as 'critical health literacy' (Nutbeam 2008). Realising one's rights typically also requires the capacity to contest authorities (Shalev, Kaplan, and Guttman 2006). In general, minority, immigrant, and economically marginalised populations are at a particular disadvantage in realising health rights because of language, cultural, and institutional barriers including discrimination (Kreps 2006; Betancourt 2007). The use of innovative and creative tools can be useful to provide marginalised communities greater control in how they wish to communicate their lived health experiences.

The next promising practice deals with the barrier of historical marginalisation and systematic discrimination. The following example illustrates the use of photo voice to support the health needs of Aboriginal women with breast cancer in Saskatchewan, Canada (Poudrier and Mac-Lean 2009). Despite some recognition that Aboriginal women who have experienced breast cancer may have unique health needs, little research has been conducted on the lived experiences of Aboriginal women.

Case study 4.4: Photovoice with Aboriginal women

The intervention aimed to make visible Aboriginal women's experiences with breast cancer using a creative technique, photovoice. The participants were Aboriginal women who had completed breast cancer treatment. The programme drew upon a critical and feminist conception of visuality to enable Aboriginal women who have experienced breast cancer to make their experiences visible in a way that recognises their experiences are situated within the structural context of marginalisation through colonial oppression. The participating women provided the initial and most important interpretations of the photos and discussed key themes extensively during interviews. The women were asked to describe the meaning of the photographs and to choose those which were most significant to them. Participants indicated two areas of priority for healthcare: (1) Aboriginal identity and traditional beliefs, although expressed in diverse ways, are an important dimension of breast cancer experiences and have relevance for healthcare; and (2) there is a need for multidimensional support which addresses larger issues of racism, power and socio-economic inequality.

The next example deals with the barrier of lack of awareness of context and resources by accounting for the disempowering conditions preventing engagement. Gender inequality and the low status of women are one of the key underlying social determinants of health in the Eastern Mediterranean region (EMR). The Basic Development Needs Programmes (Assai, Siddiqi, and Watts 2006) introduced in the EMR was carried out in poorest and rural areas with active involvement of local communities. The programme targeted gender inequality by offering loans and training to women for economic enterprises. It also included measures to improve health and well-being by providing health services, nutrition, safe water, sanitation, and shelter. The first programme was initiated in Somalia in 1988, and the model was then extended to support community development in 12 countries in the EMR: Afghanistan, Djibouti, Egypt, Iran, Iraq, Lebanon, Morocco, Oman, Pakistan, Somalia, Sudan, and Yemen. Programmes covered a population of almost three million in over 250 sites. The programmes strongly emphasised community involvement and intersectoral collaboration, facilitated by WHO linkages with ministries of health. Intervention sites were identified in response to a request from the local residents. Each village was divided into clusters of 25 to 40 households. Each cluster elected one representative, who was nominated to a village development committee. An intersectoral technical team provided training and back-up support and helped conduct a baseline survey. Each household was asked to identify their top three social development priorities. The final interventions were decided by the community on a consensus basis. WHO had a catalytic role, providing soft loans against small-scale income-generating projects and for social uplift projects such as water supply and sanitation. The experiences of two villages, Dar Mali in Atbara State, Sudan, and Gallamo in Djibouti, shows how the villagers were able to bring about the change through simple community-based interventions. Programme evaluation showed improvements in maternal care, family planning, and immunisation coverage for children and identified several strengths of the programmes including well-organised, aware, and enthusiastic communities; active participation of women in income-generating activities; empowered communities that feel confident in approaching local governments and other agencies for new projects; and better health coverage indicators.

Unequal power between service providers and communities, and the lack of ownership of communities over programmes are other important system-wide barrier to involvement of marginalised communities. In their review of community participation in South Asia, Hossain and colleagues found that community development programmes made a significant contribution to health improvement (Hossain et al 2004). They gave examples of communities involved in the planning and implementation of programmes, which facilitated the development of training and skills of community members, enabling marginalised communities to take some control over their own lives (Rifkin 2009). Here, Community Health Workers (CHW) play an important role. CHWs are lay people from a local community who are trained to deliver health interventions to that community. There is evidence that CHWs have made strong contributions to health improvements at the local level (Haines et al 2007) including reductions in maternal and child health and mortality, control of communicable diseases, such as malaria and TB, and HIV/AIDS (Lehmann and Sanders 2007). Studies report their proximity to the local communities and understanding of local cultures, contexts, and knowledge systems make them effective channels for reaching 'hard to reach' populations and improving programme uptake and impact. For instance, Cyril, Possamai-Inesedy, and Renzaho (2015) found that CHWs among minority ethnic communities improved programme feasibility and impact by enhancing the relevance of health promotion messages, fostering improved health behaviours, overcoming cultural and access barriers, and encouraging participant engagement.

The redistribution of power is a key ingredient of effective engagement with marginalised communities. This involves the redistribution of political power, economic wealth, and/or social recognition (CSDH 2008). Engaging powerholders generally takes the form of cooperative partnerships between marginalised groups and more powerful actors and agencies in health ministries, healthcare settings, development NGOs, or international research bodies (Aveling and Jovchelovitch 2014). Powerful groups seldom re-allocate health-enabling power or resources without assertive demands from marginalised people, however, which has led to the development of campaigns by marginalised communities for advancing their health rights (Campbell 2020). In asserting for this redistribution of power, marginalised communities are striving for health equity (in terms of improved health outcomes and service access). Here there are lessons from the principles and practice of community development (or community organising in the US), a process by which communities identify their assets and concerns, prioritise, and select issues, and intentionally build power and develop and implement action strategies for change (Minkler et al 2019). This attempt to redistribute power has given rise to what is known as critical public health activism, which refers to any attempt to redistribute power in ways that create more health-enabling social environments (Cowan 2021). Collective agency is seen to lie in activities by members of vulnerable groups and their allies that increase their opportunities for health and well-being. Examples include Treatment Action Campaign of South Africa and PHM (Jan Swasthya Abhiyan) in India discussed in Chapters 2 and 5 in this book.

Conclusion

This chapter has considered the experience of communities on the margins, who experience exclusion because of socio-economic disadvantage and other structural inequalities and marginal identity positions. Evidence suggests that community and rights-oriented development and participation bring a number of benefits to these marginalised communities in terms of improved health outcomes and service access. However, at the same time, there are major barriers to the engagement of marginalised communities within community participation structures and processes. The chapter has focused particularly on different aspects of promising practice in engaging these communities. There are a number of key principles underpinning this promising practice, such as improving access to health information on health rights, improving community ownership of programmes, addressing the underlying social determinants of health, and redistributing power from policy makers and service providers to local communities. It is evident that participatory processes need to be more effective at engaging marginalised communities but the inspiring examples within this chapter provide a route map for how this can be achieved.

5

Building sustainable social movements for the right to health

Introduction

The past decades have seen growing calls for public health researchers and practitioners to become more involved in politics and advocacy (Kapilashrami et al 2016). There is increased awareness of the importance of power and political determinants of health and how tackling these can generate more effective health policy (Bambra et al 2005), practice and outcomes. Yet, this interest has not percolated into mainstream debates and research on public (health) policy, which remain bereft of analysis of power and politics. There is far little engagement of public health practitioners and policy makers in proactively tackling power and political determinants of health via advocacy and activism. Such omission can be attributed to two main reasons: first, the continued dominance and resurgence of the neoliberal individual-centric Western biomedical paradigm of health in contemporary policy making and public health. This paradigm, strengthened through colonial and neo-colonial projects described earlier (Chapters 1 and 2) and advances in modern medicine, was successful in eroding holistic understandings of health and distancing states of health (and ill-health) from issues of power and politics. Second, the worlds of policy, academic research, and activism have developed in epistemic silos (Kapilashrami et al 2016). Academia and Activism are often seen as dichotomous (even if complementary) and distinct epistemic worlds that have different goals – generating knowledge and social change respectively – as well as different incentive environments and structures. The difference can be traced along the 'thinking' vs 'doing' divide that is associated with the academic and activist worlds respectively[1]. Public health and medicine on the other hand are viewed as neutral (Keshet et al 2017), concerned with the delivery of care as per standards defined by objective science, and disassociated from the politics that determines health. Against this backdrop, any calls for public health researchers and practitioners to engage with the politics of health and advocate for tackling the upstream determinants of health takes both 'practitioners and researchers beyond the traditional, evidence-based public health paradigm, raising potential dilemmas and risks for those who undertake such work' (Kapilashrami et al 2016, p 413).

The central thesis of this chapter is that advocacy and activism are essential components of public health's efforts to achieve health rights and equity, and social movements serve as critical conduits and a decisive force in this struggle for healthier societies and a fairer world.

Advocacy and activism share some commonalities. They engage people and groups to draw attention to issues of societal importance, thereby aiming to influence decision-making processes to bring about change. While advocacy focuses more on shifting attitudes and views to garner greater support for ideas or collective interests (Schmid, Bar, and Nirel 2008), activism involves more direct action that may involve challenging ideas, underlying structures, and influencing social norms and values (Smith and Ferguson 2010). Social movements involve both these processes in making change.

Starting with examining the salient features of social movements, we reflect on the critical trends in the development of social movements and the politics they espouse. We examine the theoretical developments and discuss key gaps in social movements theories. While charting scholarship on social movements, we revisit key areas of enquiry using a decolonial lens, to examine the distinction between contemporary and older movements, the place of community organising, and the politics of difference adopted by the movements of the oppressed for health rights and justice. In the latter half, the case of the People's Health Movement helps illustrate the potential of community organising and solidarity-based movements for overcoming epistemic divides to achieve health justice.

Social movements: origins, theoretical advances and deficits

Social movements are organised, non-institutional collectives that challenge 'authorities, powerholders or cultural beliefs and practices' (Goodwin and Jasper 2003). They are therefore viewed as critical for dismantling top-down power structures and bringing about social change. Premised on the assumption that the status-quo – in the case of health movements, manufactured ill-health, and gross inequities – is both undesirable and unacceptable, movements employ a range of tactics to facilitate such change. Some create opportunities for claiming new rights (for example, voting rights, rights to safe abortion) and engage with political processes. Others have responded to threats and violations with demands of restoration, compensation, and helped develop longer-term mechanisms through which public authorities can be held accountable.

Some examples of social movements include the civil rights and liberties movements and the women's movements. The feminist movement exemplifies social movements that have confronted substantial changes in the world order and made giant strides of progress on women's rights and equality via legislative, policy, and institutional changes alongside confronting societal attitudes and mind-sets. While earlier movements were organised around class and anti-colonial struggles, the twentieth century witnessed a growth in social movements organised around human rights, environmental concerns, and affirmation of difference and identities by oppressed groups (for example, caste, sexual, and queer rights).

The advent of technology and the indiscriminate use of social and digital media to organise communities and build social movements changed the nature of community organising and collective action. As a departure from classical understandings, contemporary forms of organising and movements are therefore deemed to be more informal, lacking 'clear organizational structures and internal bureaucracies, and effectively function by coalescing political identities and agendas both nationally and globally' (Thompson and Tapscott 2010, p 4).

Social movements are often conflated with activities led by the development sector via non-governmental organisations (NGOs) or charities. These are however distinct. NGOs, as also discussed in Chapter 2, are mostly project-based and target-oriented. These tend to align their priorities and activities to more centrally defined targets at global (for example, MDGs or SDGs) or national level (national plans) or reshape these based on interests of their constituencies. In contrast, social movements can be seen as more grassroots-driven, with an alternative, political vision for improving health and development. A key distinguishing feature is their foregrounding of power and politics, and utilising community organising as a political tool to effect change. They may 'bypass established development organisations, local elites and parties or engage them on different terms. But they are by no means apolitical; instead of a depoliticised development, they politicise the rights of the poor' (Escobar 1992, p 422). Realising such political vision demands confronting and dismantling of the power relations that serve the interests of the privileged class and exclude and marginalise the oppressed. Social movements play a critical role in such destabilisation of the axis of power and authority. Campaigns, another concept that is interchangeably used with social movements, are organised courses of action towards a political or social goal. They serve as critical strategies utilised by movements to coalesce around more specific demands. In health, these demands have included patent reforms to make essential medicines affordable, demanding patients' access to their medical records, disinvesting from public-private partnerships in healthcare, ending violence against women, or more specific legislative reforms that target very specific policy actors (for example, domestic violence laws to include coercive control in Scotland, inclusion of marital rape in sexual violence legislations). Because of the specificity of these demands, they are often time-bound. Social movements on the other hand take on a broader social critique, attending to the underlying determinants of these individual issues.

Scholarship and theorising of social movements have expanded over time, with 'several conceptual changes or "turns"' (Goodwin and Jasper 2003, p 5). The core questions are why and how movements arise, sustain, or fail, with considerable attention given to a range of economic, political, and cultural dimensions of social movements. In terms of *origins*, the debate has often moved between two distinct characterisations of movements. The first presents movements as spontaneous and irrational outbursts to 'structural strain on behalf of previously atomized individuals' (Crossley 2022, p 364). These spontaneous acts are led by irrational actors 'blindly following demagogues who sprang up in their midst' (Goodwin and Jasper 2009, p 5). This school of thought was predominant in the earlier writings on social movements from North America and Western Europe, focusing initially on individual grievances and on the availability and mobilisation of resources as triggers for collective action (Osaghae et al 2010). The latter part of the twentieth century saw a visible turn away from such framing, and social movements began to be seen as embedded in social networks, strategically drawing upon resources and opportunities to organise communities for collective action. Scholars examined their diverse motivations, and the various tangible and intangible *resources* that communities develop, mobilise, and draw on to effect change to their circumstances (McCarthy and Zald 1977; Tilly 1977). Other works emphasised the importance of *political context* and *systems* (including differences in the character of states) in shaping the emergence, development, and impact of social movements (Kriesi et al 1992; Kriesi 1996). An important body of work focused on '*political processes*' through which social movements interact with the State, and how these link to '*political opportunities*' generated by external environments and factors exogenous to the movement itself. These factors created incentives for collective action (Tarrow 1996, 2011). The core argument put forward was for any explanations of movement politics to consider the specificities of the national political structure and context in which social movements' organising takes place.

Critiquing the disproportionate attention to resources and political processes, other scholars drew attention to the cultural aspects in the formation of collective identities and the discursive 'frames' and how these are applied to interpret diverse issues to enable wider resonance. Benford and Snow (2000), for instance, refer to 'collective action frames' that are produced as actors negotiate a shared understanding of the problems, its determinants, and in articulating an alternative vision to affect change.

While there is a rich body of work that examines how movements come about, the analysis of social mobilisation, community organising, and action has happened largely in the context (and from the gaze) of industrial and postmodern societies, most crucially informed by the theoretical works of European and American scholars. This orientation to the analysis of movements in the Global North (Thompson and Tapscott 2010) introduces a euro-centric bias that is blinded to the longstanding tradition of organising and activism in the Global South, its particularities, and the multitude of strategies adopted.

These omissions have important implications for our understandings and future directions of study on social movements. One arena where such omission is stark is the distinction made between old and new social movements. The term 'new social movements' (NSM) is used with reference to movements that were liberated from class struggles, marking a 'shift from conflicts over material well-being to conflicts over cultural fulfilment' (Habermas 2008, p 193). These were viewed as employing new and creative forms of action and focused on identity concerns rather than on political ideology and strategy (Cohen 1985). Movements that were typically referred to as NSM were the environmental movements, women's and gay liberation, the peace movement, and cultural revolt linked to youth activism (Pichardo 1997). This distinction rests on a partial insight into environments that trigger organising around social and political concerns. Contending the basis of this distinction with reference to Latin America, Escobar (1992) observes that social movements in the South have arisen largely in response to the failed promises of colonial and postcolonial development. These therefore cannot be seen in either economic or political terms but 'within a reinterpreted context of the crisis of development and modernity' (1992, p 64). Similarly, though not rejecting the paradigm of NSMs, Ben Moussa (2013) has argued that conflicts and movements in Arab countries are still 'deeply shaped by struggles for social and economic justice'.

The lack of recognition of Southern scholarship is even more stark in the context of Islamic societies, where any form of collective action continues to be dismissed as radical outpourings on the (Arab) 'street' (Moussa 2013). Critiquing this bias and focus on religion-oriented political discourses and groups, scholars have drawn attention to the rich tradition of civil society institutions and organising in Arab countries that have historically challenged state authority and power. These include, for example, 'from trade union movements, nationalist and leftist ones, to Islamic/fundamentalist movements' (Moussa 2013, p 52). Yet, with the exception of a few recent studies (Wiktorowicz 2004; Moussa 2013), social movement theories and their contentious politics have remained devoid of Islamic activism (Wiktorowicz 2004). The 'Arab spring' – broadly referring to democratic revolutions that swept across the Middle East (starting in Tunisia) against oppressive and corrupt regimes – marked a shift in collective action within Arab countries and can be seen as a critical source for the expansion of social movement theory (Carty 2014).

In our attempts to free social movements scholarship from a colonial gaze, we identify critical gaps and distinct contributions. First, the importance of locating social movements scholarship in historical contexts and global configurations of power and capital (Amin 1993). This suggests the need for multi-level analysis to link 'the micro level of individual protesters with the meso level of social movements, and macro level of national political systems and supranational processes' (Van Stekelenburg and Klandermans 2009, p 37). Second, there is a paucity of multi-disciplinary perspectives in studying social movements. Utilising these, we emphasise the need for studying the new forms of activism as manifested in the interactions between 'collective action repertoire, new communication technologies and the politics of "recognition" and "distribution"' (Moussa 2013, p 48). The Digital revolution has facilitated collective action in diverse ways. Yet, the use of digital media for purposes of organising is often seen from an instrumental perspective. Here, the sources of connectivity and possibilities (for example, self-organising, flexible grassroots networks, transparency in action) that emerge from the use of new information and communication technology and web platforms are insufficiently examined (Carty 2014).

This chapter also develops and extends our understanding of health movements, which have hitherto been understood predominantly in the context of patients, consumers, or populations infected/affected by specific diseases. Much less exists in relation to movements that simultaneously action different societal levels – individual, community, institutional, and structural – to facilitate more long-term sustained improvements in health. Furthermore, insights and experiences of activists engaged in building social movements and their understandings of success and failures are even less prominent.

We now turn to the case of the People's Health Movement (Case Study 5.1), a prominent contemporary health movement that continues to offer a countervailing force to the ongoing threats and crisis of health. The case study offers valuable insights into holistic health movements, as distinct from disease-focused mobilisations, and the diverse strategies utilised to both build and sustain movements.

Case study 5.1: The case of the People's Health Movement

The PHM was formed in 2000, in response to failures of the international community in meeting the Health for All by 2000 goal endorsed in the Alma-Ata Declaration on Primary Health Care (1978). Since its formation, the movement has strived to develop and action, both independently and in alliance with other movements and campaigns, a global counter-hegemonic narrative on health and embolden health praxis.

Through its regional networks, country chapters, and constituent organisations working at the grassroots, the global People's Health Movement (PHM) has successfully organised health professionals, activists, human rights defenders, and grassroots as well as national organisations working with disenfranchised people in over 70 countries around its core vision of realising the right to health. The vision is supported by demands for improved access to health services and wider social, economic, and political determinants, while the movement strives to broaden the understanding of these health determinants to take cognisance of the market influences on health.

Aligned with its wide scope and political vision of Health for All, PHM activists have adopted a range of strategies and tools for activism and to build movements and affect change at local, national, and global levels. These have ranged from street protests to more organised country-level and global-level lobbying and policy advocacy projects. We describe a few of these that have affected gradual but systemic changes in policy and governance:

Community organising, people's health manifestos and their use to lobby political parties around key demands for achieving the right to health

This approach had multiple strengths and outcomes. On the one hand, the manifesto served as an effective tool to communicate key demands for health policy reforms. Multiple successes were witnessed in countries. In India, the manifesto was utilised to lobby for increase in government health spending (from 0.9 per cent to 1.2 per cent of GDP). In Scotland, political parties such as the Greens adopted the people's manifesto as the party manifesto, and PHM activists were asked to run sessions on health inequalities at party annual conferences. On the other hand, the process of developing the manifesto enabled stronger links across third sector organisations working on health issues, mobilisation of community members around Health for All goals, and their engagement with activism for improved health (for example, public hearing, human rights festival). PHM Scotland has contributed significantly to researching and campaigning for health equity in recent years, including compiling a refreshed People's Health Manifesto in 2021 and hosting a people's health inquiry on the impact of COVID-19 on health inequities in the city of Glasgow in 2022. In June 2023, the group organised a Scottish People's Health Assembly (PHA) to coincide with the global PHA taking place in Colombia at the end of the year. This involved bringing grassroots organisers and activists together to discuss synergies in fighting for health justice and trying to build a stronger health movement in the country.

Monitoring states, intergovernmental agencies, and other actors (commercial interests) has been a longstanding focus of PHM's global and national level activities

At country level, PHM activists, together with other agencies, monitor their governments' compliance with human rights regulations and make regular submissions to UN ESCR committees. These submissions are considered as 'civil society' submissions and viewed as an alternative to the government's official submission on their achievements. Besides acting as watchdogs for government policies and actions, a distinctive success of the PHM lies in its concurrent reform efforts at global level. PHM strategies are affected by a deep understanding of the importance of structural and macro-level drivers of health and well-being, and the supranational nature of governance within which health-related decision-making occurs. Thus, a core domain of action is building solidarity at international level (via people's health assemblies) and affecting change in global health governance. The latter is enabled through leading and participating in a range of civil society initiatives aimed at democratising global governance spaces. Notable among these are the WHO Watch, steering the WHO Commission for Social Determinants of Health and submissions to the FENSA process that determined WHO's position on engagement with non-State (private) actors.[2]

Innovating accountability mechanisms to hold states and providers to account and make health systems responsive

Examples of public hearings and tribunals that enabled a process of documenting violations and empowering communities to testify in front of an independent panel comprised of health experts are presented in more detail in Chapter 7 (Accountability). In some instances, these processes led to effective institutionalisation of community-based monitoring approaches. Such institutionalisation was made possible by strategic alliance and partnership with national human rights and other agencies and led to individual-level compensation as well as formulation and strengthening of grievance redressal mechanisms.

A distinctive feature of PHM has been its focus on organising and building perspectives and capacities of young activists. Recognising the need to sustain a progressive politics of health and support the creation of community-based and -led movement, PHM members have engaged in formal and informal activities to educate and empower. Most notable are the PHM's International People's Health Universities (IPHU) – held regionally and internationally – that reaches out to young activists (students, health professionals, and development practitioners) and trains them on the social, political, and commercial determinants of change and strategies for resistance. Adopting Freirean pedagogy, IPHU offers a space to learn about politics of health (raising critical consciousness) and share diverse regional and cultural experiences of activism (collectivising learnings to reshape worldviews). IPHU and the People's Health Assemblies also become the conduits for building solidarity across borders and issues, thereby offering a countervailing force to the growing individualisation of resistance.

Box 5.1: Additional references for case study

- What would it take for a paradigm shift in Scotland's health? (2023) (Scottish Left Review)
- Who will safeguard Scotland's future health? (2021) (Bella Caledonia)

- A Scottish people's health manifesto (2016)
- A people's health manifesto for Scotland (2021)
- Health inequalities in Scotland – All rhetoric, no change? (2019)
- Kapilashrami et al (2016)
- Baum, Sanders, and Narayan (2020)

Theorising health movements

Health-related movements have often been classified as NSMs (Habermas 1988), that is, mobilisations that arrived on the political stage in the latter half of the twentieth century to replace 'class-relations' and 'capitalism' as the main fault-line along which 'old' social movements were organising. Concurring with Edwards' (2004) critique of such claim, we acknowledge that such classification is based on a particular understanding of health, and that social activism on health issues have a longer, more complex and richer genealogy that go back to the nineteenth and early twentieth century. For example, labour movements' mobilisation around occupational health risks, and the women's liberation movements raising awareness and uniting over issues of reproductive control. In presenting a historical overview of the Women's Health Movement, Helen Marieskind (1975) identifies consciousness–raising collectives as critical spaces where women shared their medical experiences, recognised their lack of control over their bodies, and extended these concerns to other areas of healthcare. The self-help movements of the early 1970s (and gynaecological self-examinations) became the first transnational mobilisation around reproductive health rights and bodily autonomy, and a vehicle for a broad range of demands. These demands extended beyond reproductive rights shifting power away from institutionalised medicine and medical practitioners to feminist counter expertise, while supporting local activists (Ruault and Rundell 2016). Such collective reflection in the 1960s and 1970s coalesced around issues of reproductive control and directed to demands for a restructuring of the healthcare system and redefining healthcare.

The point regarding continuity and progression of social mobilisation and activism is also highlighted by activists engaged in the Health for All movement. In an interview-based study to gain insights into movement building, activists from Africa and Central and Latin America emphasised new movements are often offshoots of or build on 'the achievements and momentum of existing, older ones' (Musolino et al 2020, p 4), in this case, national liberation movements resisting a dictatorial or apartheid regime. The networks and knowledge derived from these struggles offered a fertile ground for the health movement to germinate.

Health movements tend to be organised around demands for (1) improving access to healthcare, often utilising the human rights lens (AAAQ framework enshrined in the General Comment 14); (2) challenging health inequities based on gender, ethnic/indigenous status, sexuality, and disability by focusing on the health rights violations and unmet needs of marginalised groups and constituencies; and (3) securing appropriate conditions for achieving the highest standards of health. The latter could range from demands for increasing public spending on healthcare and against privatisation of healthcare (for example, Keep Our NHS Public campaign) or tackling other determinants of health (for example, conflicts, forced displacement, and migration).

Brown et al (2004) identified three categories to classify health movements, noting that these are not rigid and have significant overlaps. These are: movements focusing on healthcare access and/or provision; and 'constituency-based movements' that focus on health inequalities in regard to different aspects of social location. A third category they draw attention to is 'embodied health movements' (EHM). These movements foreground embodied lived experience of specific illness/medical condition to challenge the 'science on etiology, diagnosis, treatment and prevention' and 'address disease, disability or illness experience' (Brown et al 2004). The constituents are predominantly those experiencing or affected by specific medical condition and associated stigma and discrimination. The AIDS movement is one prominent example of EHM that was significant for redefining interactions between medical or technical experts and patients or affected persons. It was perceived as not 'merely a "disease constituency" advocating for greater resource allocation and treatment but, as Steven Epstein (1996, p 8) puts it, an alternative basis of expertise' (Kapilashrami and O'Brien 2012). These movements coalesced around a shared 'identity' (in this case those living or affected by HIV) and offered a powerful counter-narrative to the biomedical and technocratic dominance in health, including questioning the power differences that define patient-provider interaction in most healthcare settings. The AIDS movement for instance fostered an unprecedented series of reforms in human rights obligations, instruments, and practices around informed consent for testing and treatment, medical confidentiality, counselling, and support to infected (and affected) individuals, to name a few (Bayer 1994). In some contexts, movements have successfully lobbied for greater transparency in decision-making, improved dignity of care, and patients having greater say in their treatment regime and control over their medical records (for example, campaign on the right to patient medical records). However, in analysing patient activism and lobbying efforts that involve disease-affected communities, caution must be exercised in understanding how they are organised, funded, and the extent to which their goals are aligned with the commercial and scientific interests vested in these. While the emergence of 'health consumer movement' (Allsop et al 2004) and Patient Advocacy Groups can be attributed to the gradual decline in patients and citizens' trust in medical professionals and other public authorities, these have also served as front organisations for drugs and other transnational commercial industries (Allsop et al 2004; Abraham 2020). Pharmaceutical companies establish or bankroll front lobbying and consumer/patient advocacy groups, cultivating a grassroots image while pushing specific drugs and treatments. We discuss this further under key issues in social movements.

A scan of existing literature on health-related social movements is telling for the emphasis given to disease-specific mobilisation and activism (for example, breast cancer, HIV/AIDS). It is unsurprising then that theoretical development has tended to focus more on resources and networks utilised in sustaining actions or examining their effectiveness from the prism of the life of these movements, and meeting of campaign demands. Much less exists on the day-to-day contestations and ethical conundrums, how activists navigate politics and power when engaging different constituencies, and the tangible and intangible outcomes and system-wide changes resulting from such mobilisation.

Processes of mobilisation and strategies employed in health movements

The People's Health Movement we described earlier adopted a two-pronged approach. First, action oriented towards empowering communities, raising awareness of their rights and strengthening 'the voice of the poor to make forceful demands' (Campbell et al 2010) to the State. Second, it works to create more receptive social environments and democratic institutions that will enable the power holders to respond to those demands. As we note in the case of the People's Health Movement described earlier, these cannot be mutually exclusive processes but synergistic actions for affecting social change.

The former focus on empowerment often involves invoking the process of 'conscientization' (Freire 1973) where safe and empowering social spaces are created to enable the oppressed and dispossessed in questioning the social roots of the problems experienced at individual or community level. However, success here can only be achieved by transcending individual-level critical reflection and dialogue to collectively developing action agendas. This process of situating the 'individual' in the 'collective' has been embedded in social movement praxis and facilitated through use of participatory action research (PAR) methods to create a community of conscious citizens. PAR methods such as community resource mapping and time-use have long been used by community development organisations and women's groups, to identify assets/resources available in the community, generate awareness of their health entitlements, and 'to align resources and policies in relation to specific system goals, strategies, and expected outcomes'. However, as several scholars emphasise, poor and disenfranchised can rarely go through this journey alone, without the support of and strategic alliances with actors and agencies that hold or effectively wield political and economic power (Nair and Campbell 2008). This brings to the fore the importance of advocacy and lobbying with institutions and actors holding political and economic power (the second of the two-prongs). Thus, the mandate for social movements goes beyond empowering the individual. Change and reform need to create environments that build the 'political capabilities of groups of poor' (Campbell et al 2010) and simultaneously sensitise and reform institutions and political actors to hear their voices and heed their demands; making them conduits between those holding power and those dispossessed of it (as depicted in Figure 5.1).

A wide range of strategies – from resistance and confrontation to cooperation and collaboration – have been adopted in bringing change at institutional and/or societal levels. These are described in more detail in the following section. Sustaining social movements, however, requires building a collective mass of activists who have a shared vision and are able to participate or engage in the strategies in varying capacities – healthcare professionals, community practitioners, human rights activists, academics. This makes 'capacity building' a cornerstone of social movements, enabling a concurrent process of individual conscientisation and building of the collective that helps broaden the base of movements and solidarity within.

The resonance of the PHM lay in health professionals successfully advocating with states and/or international bodies (WHO) on the right to health. Individuals and groups within countries helped lay the foundation for many health reforms through this advocacy. The drugs policy reforms in countries in Global South is a case in point.

Key issues in contemporary health movements

Health movements face several challenges. Studies have attributed the failure of the primary healthcare movement and its vision of Health for All by 2000 to several factors. These include the rise of neoliberalism and resulting withdrawal of State from its welfare functions, the imposition of economic austerity and structural adjustment programmes that weakened public health systems and wider determinants (such as food security). These developments paved the way for growing privatisation and dismantling of community healthcare systems (Baum et al 2016; Kapilashrami and Baru 2018; Labonté and Ruckert 2019).

Figure 5.1: Social movements as critical conduits in the struggle for right to health

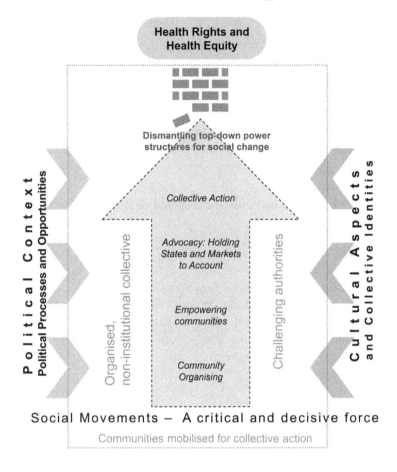

The aforementioned issues continue to pose a significant, if not greater, challenge to health activism today, stymying the gains and achievements made by past movements. For instance, the State handover of commons to the commercial sector is being aggressively pursued through Western donors and multilateral initiatives in global health (Hamer and Kapilashrami 2020).[3] Thus, a core challenge confronting organising for health rights is that the interlocutor of social movements and the right to health is the state, and demands of the movement are within a rights and accountability framework. But in most countries the infrastructure for public goods is no longer provided by the State but the markets, while the role of the state is limited to that of a manager or commissioner. This raises the question of how health movements can engage with a new accountability framework that is relevant in the context of neoliberal globalisation.

There are additional threats that health movements face today. As argued in the introduction, the most notable challenges include the shrinking spaces and resources for human rights activism amid growing conservatism, fascism, hyper-nationalism, and widening inequalities. An understanding of the challenges that activists and groups face in mobilising and sustaining collective action cannot be isolated from this macro-environment and needs to be firmly located in the social political analysis of global trends and political economy.

Against this backdrop, in the following section, we outline a few of the under-researched but critical conundrums and threats contemporary health movements face.

Neoliberalism and individualisation of resistance

The hegemony of neoliberal capitalism is identified as a critical threat to progressive struggles for health equity and justice. Much is written on what neoliberalism means for the gradual retreat of the State from its welfare functions and the impact on State-citizen relationships. However, much less is understood about how neoliberalism captures ideologies and shapes 'frameworks of thought' and 'ways of doing'. An important consequence of neoliberal thought (and the neoliberal economic system) is the individualisation of resistance and activism itself. Musolino et al (2020) draw on the theory of individualisation to discuss how alongside an increase in individual choices and freedoms, the neoliberal economic systems have led to a dis-embedding of global and national elites from national responsibilities and lessened the responsibility of the collective to the individual.

Fragmentation of civil society action spaces is a consequence of this individualisation. Rapid growth in public-private assemblages at global level (via global health initiatives) and national level (via push for increased private sector presence in healthcare and corporate social responsibility) led to the privatisation of social and political problems and changed the nature of health financing. The increased availability and reliance on project-based funding and depleting resources for advocacy generated competition and fragmented civil society spaces. This also led to a shift in organisational cultures where, Musolino et al (2020, p 11) argue: 'workers are dis-embedded from the collective, organisations are encouraged to be competitive rather than collaborative, programmes and projects are siloed, and activities are tied primarily to an economic value'.

Against this changing global political economy, a critical dilemma faced by civil society organisations and activists is whether to pursue donor-driven projects or risk closing their advocacy campaigns. Activists also experience tensions between campaigns focused on single issues (such as banning tobacco products, levying taxes on sugar, increasing affordability of drugs through patent reforms) and those addressing broader systemic and structural changes (for example, democratising global governance and increasing participation of communities in health-related decision-making, nationally and internationally).

Depoliticisation and bureaucratisation of civil society

Another effect of such fragmentation and individualisation is depoliticisation of civil society spaces and actors constituting these spaces. Scholars have discussed the developments in the 1990s, a period marked by the rise of non-government and 'third sector' organisations that were co-opted by governments and aid-agencies (Edwards 2004). This was accompanied by the growing prominence of large international NGOs, which consolidated power as recipients of health funding and key representatives in global forums. Additionally, this period saw the widespread 'trickle-down' and adoption of technical discourses on health that were successful in displacing the comprehensive 'right to health' approach that had both primary healthcare and social determinants of health at its core.

Kapilashrami (2010) in the study of the Global Fund and HIV management notes the achievements of the AIDS movement that led to the creation of the Global Fund and successful mobilisation of funds and treatment access. This critical ethnography of the PLHIV movement and implementation of the Global Fund grants in India, however, reveals the bureaucratisation of the movement, as the Fund's elite governance structures and processes 'instill a competitive environment and systematically re-configure actors around newer forms of expertise and power centres' (Kapilashrami and O'Brien 2012). Kapilashrami and O'Brien argue that institutionalisation of such activism resulted in depoliticisation of critical voices. As the PLHIV network was incorporated into the Fund organisation as 'interpretive communities' legitimising Fund's presence, its activities were made to fit with the Fund's formalised models and performance-oriented frameworks at the cost of diverting attention away from advocacy on rights violations and tackling social determinants (Kapilashrami 2020). Renee Beard (2004) similarly observes inherent biases within the mobilisation for Alzheimer disease. She notes how the movement's aims, caregivers as primary clients, and emphasis on speak-outs reproduces the same biomedical and caregiver biases that are inherent in Alzheimer's research and 'risks transforming a social movement into an interest group working for moderate reform from within existing socio-political processes and structures', rather than challenging these through political action.

Commercial interests and movement building

Several factors have contributed to such depoliticisation. Kapilashrami and Baru (2018) draw attention to the increasing blurring of boundaries between the *public* and the *private* sectors, and the health implications of the entry of commercial interests in public policy. Albeit limited, critical perspectives (as opposed to more functionalist ones) on social movements also examine the implications of such blurring for the changing nature of activism (Kapilashrami and Baru 2018), especially in the case of disease-focused mobilisations and organising. A domain where these conflicting interests are most prominent, even if sparsely documented, is Consumer and Patient Advocacy Groups. There are multiple cases where consumer and advocacy groups become intertwined with the marketing strategies of drug companies and act as front organisations for the drug industry (Lofgren 2004). For example, Impotence Australia receives funding from Pfizer and other companies to raise awareness about Viagra and similar products. Consumer and patient advocacy groups have successfully mobilised significant resources – funding and expertise – and emerged as influential actors brokering interactions between industry, governments, and patients. They also sensitise policy actors to patient interests and contribute to drug safety issues. However, Hans Lofgren (2004) highlights the risks and dilemmas associated with their incorporation into corporatist and neoliberal governance structures. He reports a highly professionalised appearance akin to business enterprises and a total lack of transparency regarding their relations with the pharmaceutical industry, including their sponsorships and proactive disclosure of possible conflicts of interest. Studies examining the influence of the pharmaceutical industry with conflicts of interest suggest that industry tends to deploy a multi-layered 'web of influence' strategy through partnerships with patient organisations (Rickard and Ozieranski 2021). These indirect types of conflicts are difficult to regulate as they are inherently hidden and rarely explicitly reported.

More contemporary theme in this discussion is the use of digital media in re-shaping the terrain of health organising and action. In Chapter 9, we describe the diverse and extensive ways in which movements utilise social and digital media to organise campaigns, disseminate information, share testimonies and lived experiences, and generate awareness of issues. Here, we focus on key issues stemming from growing digital media penetration in activism. On the one hand, digital media has provided a platform to activists to expand their reach – with communities as well as stakeholders (targets of their lobbying efforts) – and access or disseminate information at a scale previously unimagined. On the other, media serves as an exclusive forum, and one that has the ability to reframe debates and actions and confine them to those 'closely aligned with scientific and commercial interests that have sought to extract economic value from patient data' (Petersen et al 2019). Terming the alignment of contemporary patient communities with those of science and business as 'bio-digital citizenship', Alan Petersen and colleagues (2019) discuss this *shifting politics* and *enactment* of activism while analysing media and reportage generated by patient activists in two frontline movements – HIV/AIDS and breast cancer. They argue how this facilitates a shift from a struggle for rights to striving to attract more funding and improving their public profile. For example, disproportionate attention to treatments and patient data diverts attention away from the politics and insidious aspects of industry's engagement or from targeting the social determinants of the disease. Activism must be reconceptualised, they conclude, to better reflect these workings of power in the digital age.

Uneasy alliances and contested politics

The blurred boundaries between public and private via the formation of complex quasi-public-private arrangements have implications for the transparency (and conflict) of interests. A final unexplored theme is about the dilemmas and conundrums experienced by activists as they organise and build solidarity across movements and organisations with different ideologies. When forming alliances to expand the base of movements, civil society and social movement organisations (CSOs, SMOs) often confront difficult choices of whom to ally with, for what purposes and at what costs. It is essential to note that even within movements with shared goals (for example, women's rights and freedom from violence, equal opportunities, health for all), diverse ideologies may lead to divergent pathways to achieve these goals, resulting in little consensus on which is most strategic. Divergent politics and interests highlight contestations within movements, undermining any concerted efforts towards mobilisation and solidarity building, and in some cases, marking the decline of movements.

Experiences of these contestations are numerous. A prominent site of contested politics and uneasy alliance is the abortion rights movement and its evolution. The calls for safe abortion, a demand from pro-choice and pro-rights feminists, also gained traction among a section of health professionals who were seeking de-criminalisation (and de-stigmatisation of their practices) and safer medical interventions. While both groups have long shared the same goal of legalising abortion, the alliance has often been 'uneasy' and, at times, 'contradictory'.

Tracing the historical evolution of the engagement of the two communities in the context of the US, Joffe, Weitz, and Stacey (2004) identify three distinct phases in the evolving relationship between abortion supportive physicians and activists. The first phase reflects physicians' reluctance to become 'reformers' and embrace an expansive vision of abortion rights; the second involves mutual dependence marked by tensions; and the third phase features considerable accommodation between the two groups. The shift and the 'blurred roles' of physicians and lay activists (Brown et al 2004) over the past five decades have led to greater physicians' involvement in the politics of health and medicine but also more bureaucratic, professionalised feminist spaces that limit activism to medical reforms. As a result, evident tensions have emerged between the professional movement and radical feminists (Joffe, Weitz, and Stacey 2004).

Another prominent site of contestation is the activism and campaigning against *sex selective abortion practices*. These involve conducting abortions based on 'undesirable traits' such as female sex in patriarchal societies with strong son preference, congenital illness, or disabilities. Practices of selective abortions have been found in various forms in society across different countries, cultures, and jurisdictions. However, in many countries, demands for more stringent regulation of sex-selection services found resonance with and evoked support from right-wing factions and anti-abortion lobbyists. Mobilisation around sex-selection also created unease and further divisions within the feminist movement around the issue of disability. Pitting the rights to choose (pro-choice) against the right to life (pro-life), the debate on selective abortion has been a site of moral dilemma and legal conundrum among activists and a potent source of tension between women's rights and disability-rights advocates. For instance, while the feminist movement is united in its support for abortion rights on grounds of reproductive justice and women's bodily autonomy, it has been criticised by disability-rights activists for overlooking, and unwittingly legitimising, the disability bias in the implementation of selective abortion laws (such as the Prenatal Diagnostic Techniques (Regulation and Prevention of Misuse) Act 1994 or PNDT Act) (Asch 2002; Ghai and Johri 2008; Nizar 2016). While disability-rights activists do not challenge abortion laws and prenatal techniques per se, nor oppose a pro-choice perspective, they argue that the concept of individual choice is 'socially constructed and contextually located, and ... the thoughtless use of prenatal testing could reduce, rather than expand, women's choices' (Ghai and Johri 2008). They condemn the use of these techniques against foetuses with disabilities on moral, ethical, and legal grounds.

Conclusion: Charting a new agenda for social movements

This overview of social movements and organising for resistance is not exhaustive. Its purpose is to highlight historical developments and contemporary debates, particularly from a perspective that extends beyond Europe and America.

A de-colonial lens allows revisiting and challenging the assumptions regarding the objectives, genesis, and conditions that foster social movements along with the specific issues studied within social movements scholarship. Health-related movements have been dominated by a focus on diseases and drugs, and much less attention is given to movements that aspire to simultaneously improve access, systems, and wider determinants of health, and adopt strategies that go beyond lobbying and protests.

Review of current scholarship suggests that social movement theory is seriously limited in that it is based mostly on research done on movements in northern Europe and North America. Likewise, social movement practices in the Global South are under-researched. There is a need for a more granular analysis of the role social movements play in shaping agendas and creating alternative spaces for resistance and change. How do health movements identify priorities and build collective identities? What common language unites diverse strengths and transcends disciplinary and epistemic divides? What structural, societal, and individual factors support or impede movement building? These are important questions for future enquiries. Here, it is important to be mindful of the diverse interests, values, and outcomes that mediate the practice of social movements, and that not all mobilisation for common goals may lead to the development of democratic spaces and sustainable transformative change.

New developments within the field demand a more balanced approach in studying the role of both rationality and emotions. Deeper interrogation of identity politics in unique social and political contexts that movements operate in and are consequently shaped by, is needed. Most notably, and in the context of a contemporary globalised yet atomised society, a critical question for social movements scholars and activists is how and under what circumstances local level organising and action 'moves up', and global organising finds traction in remote local contexts.

6

Addressing political, economic, and commercial forces shaping health

Cochabamba, a city in Bolivia, was the site of fierce protests against the rise in prices of drinking water in the early months of 2000. The story of the Cochabamba Water War provides a unique example of how communities came together to successfully resist the routine prescriptions of the neoliberal development model (Assies 2003).

Cochabamba had been facing an acute shortage of potable water for a long time and despite drilling deep wells, the problem kept recurring. The issue of drinking water had become a matter of serious concern for residents and several protests were organised throughout the 1990s. In September 1999 the government signed a contract for privatisation of water supply through *Aguas del Tunari*, a consortium of British, Spanish, and American companies. A special law, Law 2029 on Potable Water and Sewerage, was enacted earlier to make this possible (Assies 2003). The local College of Engineers estimated that this would result in price hikes of up to 180 per cent for poorer populations. Soon a local protest committee was formed that included engineers and other professionals as well as trade unions. In January 2000, the first set of bills with much higher rates were dispatched. The citizens were dismayed and protested. The water supply company threatened to cut off the supplies. On 11 January 2000, the coordination committee called for a 24-hour civic strike. Negotiations started with the company and the government and continued till March. Between 4 and 7 April a series of marches and strikes was organised, and the government responded with tear gas and arrests. One student was killed. On 8 April, the president announced a State of Emergency, but the protests spread to other cities (Assies 2003).

What was happening in Cochabamba had roots in decisions taken elsewhere. The World Bank had earlier entered the arena of healthcare through its 1987 policy paper, Financing Health Services in Developing Countries: An Agenda for Reform. The core argument of this push for policy reform was that governments should reduce spending on high-cost healthcare services and limit their resources to essential health services like immunisation for the poor. The privatisation of public services like water was part of the conditions that Bolivia had to agree to for a 138 million

USD loan from the International Monetary Fund in 1998. In 1999, the World Bank, in a public expenditure review for Bolivia, had encouraged 'no subsidies should be given to ameliorate the increase in water tariffs in Cochabamba' (Gonzalez and McCarthy 1999). Commenting on the protests in Bolivia on 12 April, the then World Bank President James Wolfensohn defended the rise in water charges saying that the 'biggest problem with water is the waste of water through lack of charging'. This led to a huge protest against the World Bank and the International Monetary Fund (IMF) in Washington DC (Frontline World 2002). Before the end of the month the law was revised and moves to privatise water were reversed.

Water is one of the key determinants of good health, and the supply of clean potable and uncontaminated water is an essential public service. The example earlier shows how healthcare and other health maintaining and enhancing services are shaped by global institutions, policies, economic trends, and national politics. These 'upstream' forces, referred to as the economic and political determinants of health, affect the downstream factors shaping people's health and societies.

The idea that inequalities in society are strongly related to health of communities was highlighted by the WHO Commission on Social Determinants of Health (CSDH 2008). The report highlighted how societal inequalities, including norms and practices which promoted or tolerated the unfair distribution of resources, wealth, and power, affected the daily lives of people and in turn their health. These conditions of daily living that included access to food, water, sanitation, safe housing, as well as decent work, affected people's ability to live healthy lives or to secure appropriate healthcare services.

This chapter attends to these powerful economic, political, environmental, and commercial determinants of health, their growing salience in the struggle for health rights and how civil society and social movements have attempted to promote and protect these rights. The chapter also discusses some of the challenges emerging from the interaction of economic, social, and political forces in contemporary times, and their implications for struggles for health rights.

Political determinants, globalisation, and the struggles for the right to health

Health is a political choice, and politics is a continuous struggle for power among competing interests. (Kickbusch 2015)

This assertion from Ilona Kickbusch, a political scientist at the Graduate Institute for Health and Development Studies at Geneva, in an editorial in *The British Medical Journal* (2015) encapsulated the now common wisdom that health is determined by factors beyond the individual. It signals the growing recognition by the international community and global agencies like the WHO and the World Bank that health is connected with political choices, in matters relating to how health and allied systems are financed and governed both at the country level and internationally (Ruger 2007). Attending to health therefore demands attention to these forces, and an assessment of how 'different power constellations, institutions, processes, interests, and ideological positions' (Kickbusch 2015, p 1) affect people, societies, and the structural conditions of daily living. These conditions include poor environment, unsafe water and neighbourhoods, poor and insecure housing, inadequate nutrition and harmful foods, and affect health across different political systems and cultures.

The struggles in Cochabamba described at the outset evidence an erosion of enabling conditions, but also highlight that poor and marginalised populations are no longer passive observers willing to accept these injustices. They are actively resisting the drivers of inequities.

The Lancet Commission on Political Determinants of Health in its 2014 report captured the abysmal status of these conditions and resulting states of ill-health and failed development. It noted:

- About 842 million people worldwide are chronically hungry, one in six children in developing countries is underweight, and more than a third of deaths among children younger than five years are attributable to malnutrition.
- Life expectancy differs by 21 years between the highest-ranking and lowest-ranking countries on the human development index. Even in 18 of the 26 countries with the largest reductions in child deaths during the past decade, the difference in mortality is increasing between the least and most deprived quintiles of children.
- More than 80 per cent of the world's population is not covered by adequate social protection arrangements. In 2012, global unemployment rose to 197.3 million, indicating 28.4 million increase from 2007. Wage inequalities are staggering. More than 60 per cent of workers in southeast Asia and Sub-Saharan Africa earn less than $2 per day.
- Many of the 300 million Indigenous people face discrimination, which hinders them from meeting their daily needs and voicing their claims. Girls and women face barriers to access education and secure employment compared with boys and men, and women worldwide still face inequalities with respect to reproductive and sexual health rights. These barriers diminish their control over their own life circumstances.

These abysmal health states are not merely an outcome of genetics or unhealthy behaviours/lifestyles but an outcome of systematic process of 'structuring relationships, distributing resources and administering power' that shape conditions and opportunities for either advancing or worsening health inequity (Dawes 2020, p 44). This process, which we understand as the political determination of health, involves decades of unhealthy policy choices and governance (re)structuring that introduced power asymmetries with significant consequences for poor countries and populations.

The ability of LMICs to make adequate investments for essential public services and guarantee access to key determinants was severely constrained after the IMF and the World Bank made their loans to these countries conditional upon their reducing public sector spending and privatising public services. The 'Washington Consensus' of 1989 and associated 'structural adjustments' proposed that countries not only reduce public spending but also liberalise and privatise their economies. This promoted the era of neoliberal globalisation and trade liberalisation that granted multinational corporations greater access to markets all over the world through free market bilateral and regional agreements like the North American Free Trade Agreement (NAFTA) in 1994 and institutions such as the World Trade Organization (WTO) in 1995.

The increasing dominance of the free market logic, corporate interests and profit motivation are key elements of neoliberal globalisation. The overall size of the global economy grew, and the cost of goods also came down as companies shifted production to cheaper locations. However, economic globalisation also led to impoverishment as well as deepening inequalities. Ravindran (2014) argues that economic liberalisation and fiscal discipline have not only reduced governments' expenditures but by reducing tariffs and taxes has also affected their overall revenues. Reduced public expenditure has adversely affected the lives of the poor. A study on the privatisation of water in different Latin American countries found that even in countries where more families got access to water (such as Argentina), the gains were disproportionately greater for higher- and middle-income families (Mulreany et al 2006). The authors concluded that 'water privatization represents a troubling shift away from the conception of water as a good requiring common social management, and towards the conception of water and water management services as commodities that individuals can purchase as they can afford' ((Mulreany et al 2006, p 29). Trade liberalisation in agriculture through GATTS had significant consequences. Increased dependency on food imports and declining sovereignty, increased volatility of food prices due to the introduction of 'markets' and speculative trading has led to a rise in reports of increased food insecurity, especially in LMICs. In Asia food prices that were relatively stable in the 1990s kept rising subsequently thereafter (Ambrose 2005). This contributed to increasing impoverishment, income inequality, and malnutrition directly affecting the health of the poor.

Health services were one of the key sectors affected. Hunyen, Martens, and Hilderink (2005) have suggested a multi-nature, multi-level conceptual framework to explain how globalisation affected the health of people. Changes in global governance structures and introduction of market mechanisms had profound effects on health services. 'Health sector reforms' introduced in the 1990s increased privatisation of healthcare and social services, instituted user fees, and expanded health insurance. Privatisation of healthcare services continues to be an ongoing policy thrust in countries across the world, albeit at a different pace and intensity. In Europe, where there was a strong tradition of socialised healthcare, privatisation was introduced in different ways. In the UK, the National Health Service (NHS) was established after World War II to ensure that healthcare was available to everyone. However, during Margaret Thatcher's tenure as prime minister, privatisation took place by contracting the private sector to deliver certain services, with the government covering the costs. In Belgium, an increasing proportion of hospital costs are being paid by patients. In Germany, there has been privatisation of healthcare service provision with an increasing proportion of for-profit providers (Maarse 2006).

Contrary to the theoretical assumptions behind structural adjustments and health sector reforms, there is mounting evidence to suggest detrimental effects on access, utilisation, and wider health systems. Studies report that user fee, cost recovery mechanisms, and introduction of markets through insurance resulted in reduced utilisation of services for critical conditions and diseases and increased catastrophic health spending (Gilson and Mills 1995). Growing inequities were observed as insurance schemes covered only a small proportion of the population who were formally employed, and a sizeable portion of the government subsidies benefited civil servants (Gilson and Mills 1995).

While the era of health sector reforms facilitated a greater role of markets in healthcare, the setting of the Millennium Development Goals (MDGs) consolidated the vertical approach to health systems and the private sector's presence in health. Maternal and child health were important outcome indicators for the MDGs. A review of the effect of structural adjustment programmes on maternal and children's health published in 2017 included 13 studies which studied loans from IMF, WB, and the African Development Fund, and their impact on maternal and child health outcomes in countries (Thomson, Kentikelenis, and Stubbs 2017). Some of these studies included 30 or more African countries while others included up to 82 developing countries in different parts of the world. While no study reported clear benefits, eight of the ten studies related to infant or child mortality and all three studies on maternal mortality showed that the structural adjustments had a detrimental effect. The authors concluded: 'the almost unanimous identification of a detrimental effect among existing studies ought to compel the IFIs (International Financial Institutions) to acknowledge and address health and social indicators in a much more systematic manner'. It is not surprising that only a handful of countries were successful in meeting both the maternal and child health targets of the MDGs (Countdown to 2030 n.d.).

Effects of globalisation on poverty and inequality

Many proponents of neoliberal globalisation point out that in the years since it has been promoted, the total number of poor in the world has reduced. The World Development Report of 2001, titled *Attacking Poverty*, provides interesting contrasts among countries in terms of poverty and inequality (World Bank 2001). While the overall share of the world's population living on less than $1 a day fell from 28 per cent to 24 per cent, this decline was due to reduction of poverty in East Asia or primarily China. In Europe and Central Asia, countries that were transitioning from socialism to capitalism, the number of people living on less than $1 a day rose more than twentyfold. South Asia and Sub-Saharan Africa, two of the poorest regions in the world, saw a very high rise in the number of the very poor during this period. The report also acknowledges that even though there have been many gains in terms of wealth, capabilities, and connections, the distribution of these gains is 'extraordinarily unequal'.

The concept of poverty has also undergone changes in recent years. It is no longer restricted to a 'physiological model of deprivation' limited to income or consumption and a focus on basic material or biological needs. It is being increasingly understood through the 'social model of deprivation' that includes elements like lack of autonomy or powerlessness, lack of respect or dignity, human rights, vulnerability, and inequality (Shaeffer 2008). Vulnerability in this context indicates the risk or likelihood of falling into poverty when exposed to stress or pressure. Inequality is no longer about the average levels of income or consumption of an entire population but its distribution among those people.

There is a growing interest in inequality and its relationship with poverty. According to Ravallion (1997), if levels of inequality are very high to begin with, then it is possible that despite high growth, poverty can increase. The World Inequality Report 2022 highlights that the overall inequality within countries has risen compared to inequality between countries (Chancel et al 2022). It adds that the choices made by leaders have made nations poorer, while a small proportion of individuals have become extremely wealthy. These choices as described earlier include growing privatisation of public goods, cuts to public spending in welfare services, and neoliberal reforms in the health sector. The increasing impoverishment of nations has clear implications on the ability of the state to provide public services like healthcare, food security, safe water, sanitation, or basic education which are essential for the poor.

The Lancet – University of Oslo Commission on Global Governance in Health (2014) start their report with the key message that 'the unacceptable health inequities within and between countries cannot be addressed within the health sector, by technical measures, or at the national level alone, but require global political solutions' (Ottersen et al 2014). The rising inequalities in health are a result of several factors that are beyond the control of nations and include transnational corporations as well as civil society and others. The report acknowledges that though the poorest populations in the poorest countries face the highest health risk, this is not due to poverty but a result of socio-economic inequality. It reiterated what other researchers had asserted earlier – that the more unequal a society, the poorer are its outcomes. It identifies power asymmetries as the root cause of inequality.

Pushback against neoliberal reforms and economic globalisation

While structural adjustments were supposed to lift poor nations out of poverty, they ended up becoming routes for poor nations to supply cheap labour for the global manufacturers and markets for the global economy (Debt Data Portal n.d.). Many countries went into and continue to be in deep debt, and a significant portion of national budgets continue to go into debt servicing (Abbasi 1999).

The growing debt crisis catalysed the emergence of people's networks and social movements from the 1980s onwards with demands of debt cancellation and relief (Figure 6.1). Demonstrations started being organised at World Bank and IMF meetings. In the 1990s the Jubilee 2000 campaign, with its headquarters in the UK, mobilised millions of people around the world in support of the campaign goals (Collins 1999). The Jubilee South coalition was formed, as the name suggests, in the countries of the Global South and focused on awareness generation and mobilisation for debt cancellation (*Global Call to Action Against Poverty (GCAP) – People Rising to End Inequalities* n.d.). The movement strengthened as newer campaigns were launched in the past decade. For example, the #CancelTheDebt or the UK-focused #ResetTheDebt campaigns. These highlight the persistence of debt crisis and the increase in the number of LMICs witnessing such crisis, which more than doubled since 2015 (from 22 to 55 LMICs). These countries are now facing significant poverty burdens, and difficulties providing essential public services. The global campaign was successful in making external indebtedness a high politics issue in multilateral policy debates, and ultimately led to the writing-off of more than USD100 billion of debt owed by the poorest countries. Debt relief strategies are complemented by powerful campaigns focused on raising taxes from companies profiteering from health and climate crisis. The Robinhood tax campaign is one such idea. Embodying a redistributive intent, the campaign calls for a small tax on financial transactions to tackle poverty and climate change. A similar proposal was mooted to levy a windfall tax on excess profits made by companies that benefited from a change in consumption patterns digital/online retail brands) or testing and other pharmaceutical companies (Azémar et al 2022).

The movement against global debt and poverty used popular media including rock concerts and celebrity endorsements to draw attention to the issue. The well-known 'Make Poverty History' campaign is a prime example. Bono from the rock-band U2 is one of the global champions on this issue. Currently, the Global Coalition Against Poverty, a Southern-led network, is one of the largest global networks working on issues of inequality, poverty, and human rights with 58 national coalitions across

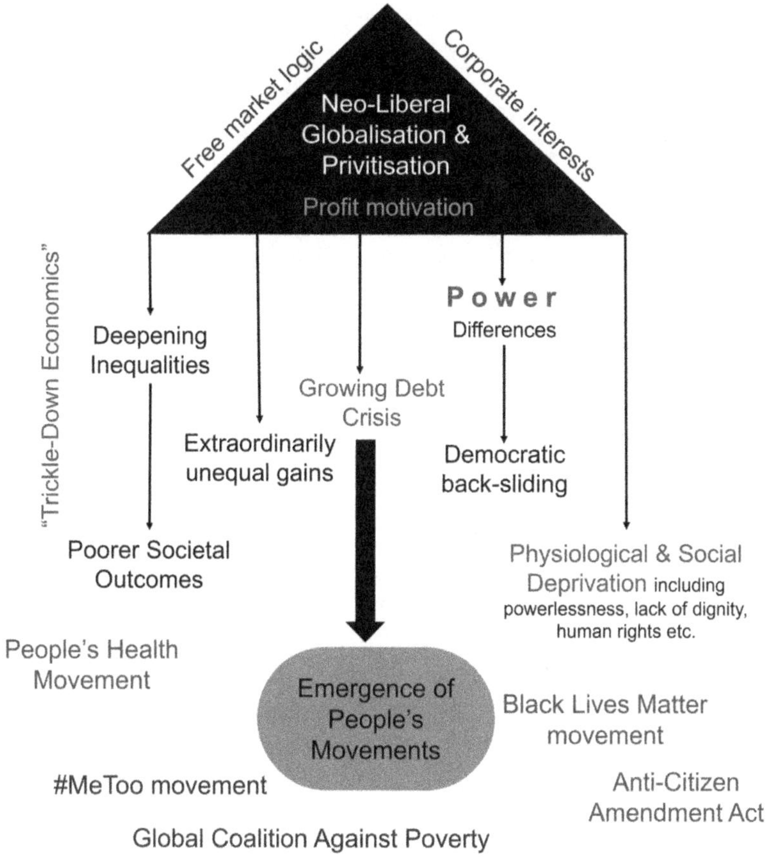

Figure 6.1: Effects of neoliberal globalisation – emergence of community movements

the world (Hunyen, Martens, and Hilderink 2005). Raising awareness and drawing attention of policy makers and the wider public to the deleterious impacts of economic globalisation on health has been a core objective of health activism. We described the organic and grassroots origins of the People's Health Movement (PHM) in Chapter 2. Since the first People's Health Assembly in Savar, Bangladesh in 2000, the PHM and its country members have launched initiatives and organised campaigns. Country-level action have been taken by members in Spain, Italy, Philippines, India, Brazil, South Africa, Columbia, DRC, and others (Bodini, Sanders, and Sengupta 2018; Nandi, Vracar, and Pachhauli 2020), focusing on the impacts on health systems and access to essential medicines.

The PHM, with other allies such as Medact and Third World Network, published five editions of the Global Health Watch report analysing the contemporary political, economic, and social determinants of health. Particular attention is given to the role of powerful institutions such as the WTO, IFC, and other regional blocks, highlighting how trade and other policy regimes are impacting population health. We describe some of these effects and actions later in this chapter.

Targeting the democratic deficit in the global health governance structures, PHM also engages with WHO through the WHO Watch, preparing detailed critiques of WHO policies and actions, and influencing its engagement with non-state actors (through the FENSA process). PHM members also attend WHO convened events raising these concerns (Baum, Sanders, and Narayan 2020).

Though all countries are considered equal on international platforms, there are vast power differences between poor and rich nations. This asymmetry extends into the donor-recipient relationships that are inherent in development aid practices. However, states also have diminishing power in the global arena as transnational corporations have emerged as extremely powerful players not only because of their economic clout but because they can easily avoid regulation by state authorities by shifting operations and jurisdictions. These transnational corporations affect the health of people in multiple ways, including poor wages and working conditions, environmental pollution, and often through the harmful goods they produce which include tobacco, sugary beverages, or fast/processed food.

Commercial determinants of health

There is a growing interest in the health impacts of the actions (and inactions) of the commercial sector. A groundbreaking report from the WHO European region on non-communicable diseases (WHO 2024b) found that the products of just four industries – fossil fuels, alcohol, ultra processed food, and tobacco – together account for at least a third of the

Figure 6.2: Health inequalities and determinants

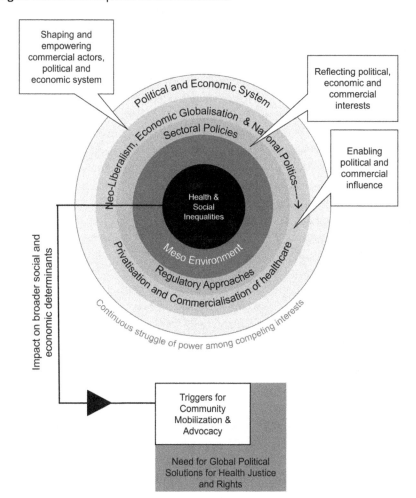

global deaths each year and likely far more with many of these occurring prematurely. The report calls for robust regulation and financial reforms to limit industry power and protect public health, and for public health actors to develop competencies in economic and legal frameworks, enforce transparency, and manage conflicts of interest effectively.

This does not account for the large burden of preventable communicable diseases and deaths that result from commercial practices. The 'systems, practices, and pathways through which commercial actors drive health and equity' (Gilmore et al 2023) are collectively referred to as the commercial determinants of health (CDoH). These determinants can shape environments and behaviours, leading to health risks and poor outcomes. Direct pathways of influence include production and distribution of drugs and medical devices, provision of services, as well as the aggressive marketing strategies (branding, promotions) that shape public perceptions and behaviours. The global Commercial Healthcare Distribution Market was valued at USD 7,074 million in 2023 and is expected to grow to USD 10,520 million by 2030. Additionally, commercial actors can indirectly affect health by influencing policies, norms, and governance that are favourable to industries and can worsen their impact on health. Commercial actors also shape knowledge and policy by funding biased research or spreading misinformation (Maani et al 2021).

Although commercial practices and interests are now receiving attention at global level (as evident from the ongoing systematic review by the WHO and Lancet Commission), these have been core to health activism since decades. Activists have long called out and resisted harmful marketing of products like breastmilk substitutes and tobacco, industrial emissions, as well as unethical practices in the fertility industry and by commercial healthcare providers.

Tobacco control and smoking cessation provide a very visible example of health advocacy and public pushback against the corporate sector for health-related reasons. Not long ago, smoking was seen as a symbol of modernity, very publicly visible and often celebrated. Consistent advocacy and litigation against tobacco companies, drawing upon evidence on the adverse impact of smoking on health and the aggressive marketing practices of tobacco giants, changed public perception and introduced groundbreaking regulatory practices at a global level. The Framework Convention on Tobacco Control (FCTC) is a prime example of successful global health governance, providing a strong regulatory framework. It also highlights the power of transnational advocacy, as its creation was largely driven by civil society activism (Mamudu and Glantz 2009). Today, smoking is widely recognised as harmful, even by smokers themselves. Many countries have banned or restricted smoking in public places, and tobacco sales are regulated. However, despite overwhelming evidence against smoking, tobacco companies continue to find new ways and markets to promote their products (Hoe et al 2022), underscoring the ongoing need for vigilance and innovative counter strategies for regulating commercial actors.

The Pharma Industry and Health – The corporate imperative of profit before people, and its underlying political support, came into sharp focus during the struggle to make anti-retroviral treatment widely available. In the early 1990s the US Food and Drug Administration (FDA) started approving antiviral drugs which were successful in halting the progress of AIDS. By 1997, AIDS-related deaths had reduced considerably in the US. However, these drugs were extremely expensive. For example, Highly Active Anti-Retroviral Therapy (HAART) using multiple drugs cost up to USD 1000 per month. South Africa had the highest HIV/AIDS infection rates in the world and needed a cheaper supply of anti-retroviral drugs for its public sector. The patents for these drugs were held by the US drug companies who would not negotiate lower prices. Reference has already been made to the Treatment Action Campaign (TAC) of South Africa and transnational activism against restrictive patent regimes in earlier chapters. The South African government, under pressure from TAC, passed a law to import these drugs from other sources. The pharma industry challenged the constitutionality of this law in the High Court of South Africa. The South African Government argued that the law complied with TRIPS (Trade Related Intellectual Property Rights) flexibilities which allowed for parallel imports and compulsory licensing.

The US pharmaceutical industry vigorously opposed this new amendment and put the South African Government and South Africa on the Special 301 'watch list' which is the step before announcing trade sanctions. This attracted a lot of media attention in the US. US-based AIDS activists targeted Vice President Al Gore, the then co-Chair of the US South African Binational Commission, during his presidential campaign. The US Congress held hearings on the role of the US Government in tackling the global HIV/AIDS epidemic. In September 1999 South Africa was removed from the Special 301 'watch list' and the prices of anti-retroviral drugs made by US companies were reduced drastically (Wadman 1999). A similar situation occurred in Brazil, where the government confronted both the US pharmaceutical industry and the US government. Brazil utilised various global platforms, such as the UN Commissioner on Human Rights (UNCHR), the World Health Assembly (WHA), and the UN General Assembly Special Session (UNGASS) on HIV and AIDS, to connect human rights with access to medicines. Over time, Brazil not only ensured free treatment access but also helped build global consensus to reduce the prices of AIDS drugs (Nunn, Fonseca, and Gruskin 2009).

The TRIPS Agreement under which the US pharma industry was trying to stall the access of cheap medicine for AIDS patients in South Africa and Brazil is a multilateral WTO agreement related to patents and transfer of technology. Drug patents have been a powerful tool to protect commercial interests, and patent regimes and their applications have undermined access to medicines for large parts of the world.

One example relates to the anti-cancer drug 'imantinib mesylate' and its production and sale in India. When India signed on to TRIPS in 1995, it was bound to change its patent regime to a 'product' patent regime within 10 years. At that time India had a 'process' patent regime which allowed Indian generic pharma companies to produce many new and patented drugs through alternative pharmacological processes. Indian companies were thus able to sell many expensive medicines at a fraction of their price elsewhere. The availability of cheap Indian anti-retrovirals was one of the reasons US pharma companies had to relent in the case of South Africa.

After India introduced a product patent regime, the Swiss pharmaceutical giant Novartis filed a patent for a new version of its drug Glivec. However, a much cheaper generic version of the drug, imatinib, was already available in India. In 2006, the Indian patents office rejected Novartis' application, calling it an attempt to 'evergreen' or extend patents through minor modifications. Novartis first appealed to the Madras High Court, which rejected their appeal. Several Indian and international health groups, such as OXFAM and Médecins Sans Frontières (MSF), urged Novartis to drop the case, and legislators in Europe and the US wrote open letters to the Novartis CEO with the same request (*Novartis Angers Critics in India, MSF* n.d.). Students and AIDS activists also protested in the US. Meanwhile, Novartis filed an appeal in the Supreme Court of India, challenging the rejection of their patent application. In April 2013, the Supreme Court ruled against Novartis, a decision praised by experts and activists for improving access to affordable medicines.

The issue of drugs patents and unequal access to healthcare became starkly evident during the COVID-19 pandemic. The pandemic was marked by a significant gap in vaccine distribution and access between high and low- and middle-income counties, what is also referred to as 'vaccine apartheid'. The pandemic's severity led states to support vaccine production in various ways, including funding research, easing regulatory hurdles, and purchasing vaccines in bulk. Despite these efforts, disparities in vaccine access persisted, underscoring ongoing global inequalities in healthcare. Transnational pharmaceutical companies and high-income countries, where such companies are based, have opposed patent waivers, and blocked generic vaccines.

The widespread advocacy around right to vaccines led to the COVID-19 Vaccines Global Access Facility (COVAX), which was established to ensure equitable vaccine access to all, but has failed to deliver. Large sections of people in Sub Saharan Africa remain unvaccinated (Bajaj, Maki, and Stanford 2022). COVAX is coordinated by WHO along with Gavi – the Vaccine Alliance and CEPI (Coalition for Epidemic Preparedness and Innovations), both of which are global health initiatives funded primarily by a private philanthropy Bill and Melinda Gates Foundation (BMGF). The coordination mechanism includes pharma companies and vaccine manufacturers but has no representation from countries which are the expected beneficiaries, scientists, or patient bodies. Despite promising cost containment due to its potential for large-scale purchase of vaccine, COVAX ended up paying higher costs for the vaccines (PHM 2021). Even after receiving considerable public funding, vaccine manufacturers ended up making unforeseen profits, and the countries depending upon COVAX faced huge shortfalls of vaccines (Pilkington, Keestra, and Hill 2022).

Countering the rise of vaccine nationalism that delayed access to vaccination in many LMICs, activists and organisations united under the People's Vaccine

Alliance coalition. The coalition was aimed at campaigning for a 'people's vaccine' for COVID-19 that is based on shared knowledge and is freely available to all, irrespective of their location. The coalition organised the Global Day of Action to End Vaccine Apartheid. Over 100 organisations and network members in 33 countries took part calling EU leaders to support TRIPPS waiver proposals and other actions to demand pharma companies accountable. The coalition has since re-branded itself to focus on people's medicines – medicines that are being developed with public funding.

Health activists also called for removal of pharmaceutical monopolies on COVID-19 tests, vaccines, and treatments. Recognising the limits of the covax facility, they demanded a policy platform to promote more equitable roll-out of vaccines, support the expansion of local production of vaccines by technology transfer and an immediate waiver of key provisions of the TRIPS Agreement (Legge and Kim 2021). Advocacy efforts focused on greater international cooperation for redistribution and increasing manufacturing capacity in the Global South.

Facing the challenge of the environmental determinants of health

Today, discussions on carbon footprints and climate change dominate conversations, but this has not always been so. In 1962, when Rachel Carson published 'Silent Spring' highlighting the impact of pesticides on the environment and human health, there was a great furore. The chemical industry funded a campaign to discredit her and the book. She was called an 'alarmist' and described as an 'ignorant and hysterical woman who wanted to turn the earth over to the insects' (Raksin 1987). In 1964 she died of cancer, but her book had become a best-seller and caught the imagination of the public and the political establishment. President John F. Kennedy ordered an investigation that led to tightening of regulations regarding the use of pesticides. While pesticide regulations were strengthened in much of North America and Western Europe, they continued to be much laxer elsewhere – in poorer countries of the world. These were exploited by industry resulting in the widespread practice of 'pesticide dumping'.

On the night of 2 December 1984, a gas leak took place in the Union Carbide pesticide factory in Bhopal, a city in India. Forty tons of deadly gas methyl isocyanate, an intermediate in the production of the pesticide Sevin, leaked from a storage tank due to a malfunction resulting from poor maintenance. Thousands died on that night itself and a further 15,000 to 20,000 premature deaths have been attributed to the leak (Broughton 2005). Hundreds of thousands were maimed and continue to suffer long-term health consequences including cancer and congenital conditions, making it the world's worst industrial disaster. The Union Carbide Corporation responded by shifting blame to a potential sabotage. They avoided being litigated in US courts where they would face huge liability and offered a settlement of 470 million USD in 1989.

Affected communities or 'survivors of the disaster' along with human rights and other organisations have led a robust campaign highlighting the injustice and used a range of tactics to seek compensation from those responsible for the disaster. The Government of India enacted a Bhopal Gas Leak Disaster Act to support survivors, but survivors' organisations assert that the support has been inadequate. These organisations organised demonstrations against inadequate relief and care and took legal recourse to seek compensation and medical care for the affected communities. Four decades later, survivor organisations, like the *Bhopal Gas Peedit Mahila Purush Sangharsh Morcha* and Bhopal Group for Information & Action, along with human and environmental rights activists, continue to demand justice and adequate compensation (The Indian Express 2021; Amnesty International 2024). A core part of this justice campaign was to expose complicity of the US and Indian governments, the former repeatedly intervening to protect the American corporate giant Union Carbide, and subsequently its new owner – Dow Chemicals – from legal liability (Burke 2019). Engaging in shareholder activism, and through representations in the UK parliament, survivor organisations continue to urge shareholders and investors (for example, Royal Bank of Scotland) to disinvest from Dow Chemicals.

Climate change and environmental activism

The world is at a different moment now with regards to environmental activism. Climate change is considered among the most burning concerns facing the planet today. The UN Environmental Program (UNEP) and the World Meteorological Organisation (WMO) had set up the Intergovernmental Panel on Climate Change which in 2013 concluded that climate change was not only real but was a result of human activities notably the release of polluting gases from burning fossil fuels. The average temperature of the world is inexorably soaring as a result of climate change. Ice caps are melting, and the sea levels are rising. The consequences include extreme weather events like storms, droughts, loss of species. But it also affect human lives through displacement, affecting both food production and health. See Figure 6.3 for an infographic of climate-sensitive health risks, vulnerabilities, and exposure pathways.

While there is considerable agreement on why there is climate change, there are still several disagreements on how climate change could be slowed and halted. The UN processes have taken a lead through a series of conferences over the years. On 13 November 2021, the 26th UN Climate Change Conference concluded in Glasgow with the adoption of the Glasgow Climate Pact.

Figure 6.3: Health and climate change

"The burning of fossil fuels is killing us. Climate change is the single biggest health threat facing humanity. While no one is safe from the health impacts of climate change, they are disproportionately felt by the most vulnerable and disadvantaged."

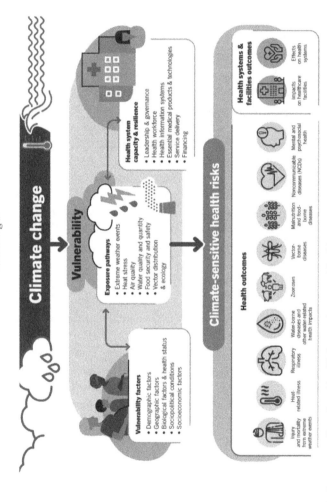

Source: https://www.who.Int/news-room/fact-sheet/detail/climate-change-and-health

Following up on the earlier Kyoto Protocol in 1997 and the Paris Agreement in 2015, the Glasgow Pact was an attempt to get countries across the world to reinforce their commitments to reduce their carbon emissions and climate action. While there is increasing evidence that global warming is leading to catastrophic climate change across the world, there are many challenges to reaching the targets that have been set in reducing greenhouse gas emissions. One of the key debates between industrialised and post-industrial nations of the Global North and the countries in the Global South relates to a country's overall contribution to greenhouse gases and who will bear the costs of mitigation. Richer countries like the US, Canada, Australia, and those in Western Europe have contributed to nearly half of all historical emissions and continue to have much higher per capita emissions. However, the impacts and burden of climate change are borne more acutely by poorer nations and most marginalised populations (for example, Indigenous groups). Many of these nations are at varying stages of development and production capacities and are relying on fossil fuels to grow their economies and improve the overall standards of living.

Despite the overwhelming evidence of the contribution of the United States to greenhouse gases there is a steadfast denial by many influential people in business and politics, especially in the US, that climate change is a result of human activities. Gregory Wrightstone, CEO of CO_2 Coalition, an advocacy organisation funded by such businesses, wrote in a recent blog: 'the claim that most modern warming is attributable to human activities is scientifically insupportable. The truth is that we do not know' (CO2Coalition 2021). Forty-four such organisations thanked President Trump in 2017 for withdrawing from the Paris Agreement on reducing greenhouse gases (Competitive Enterprise Institute et al 2017). Many of these organisations are think-tanks funded by US corporations. According to research by Influence Map, a think-tank investigating the impact of big business on climate change, the eight largest publicly traded oil and gas majors invested over 1 billion USD on misleading the public on their actions to mitigate climate change in the three years following the Paris Agreement (Laville 2019). Many companies are said to resort to 'greenwashing' or providing false or misleading information that its products and activities are environmentally safe or sustainable. Several corporations have been pulled up for running greenwashing campaigns (Robinson 2022). These corporate tactics and their narratives for misleading the public mirror those used by the tobacco industry (Lawrence 2019; Supran and Oreskes 2021), including use of same researchers and public relations firms (Hulac 2016).

The need for climate action has long been the call of environmentalists. One of the earliest and most iconic expressions of environmental activism was the Greenpeace ship Rainbow Warrior which led anti-whaling, anti-seal hunting, and even anti-nuclear testing protests at sea. In 1985, Rainbow Warrior was sunk by operatives of the French Intelligence Agency in Auckland in New Zealand, while protesting French anti-nuclear tests.

Environmental activism benefited from the synergies between different movements and communities, with health workers playing a critical role in bridging the gap between clinical practice, research, and street activism. The interconnectedness of environment, health, and peace was acknowledged and translated into activism as early as 1980 in the founding of the International Physicians for the Prevention of Nuclear War (IPPNW). Countering the Cold War divisions in the world, physicians united across the two military blocks and organised themselves around a growing movement of health for peace. The objective was to sound a medical warning to humanity about the seriousness and lethality of nuclear war and disinvest from and ban nuclear arms.

Throughout the 1980s and the 1990s, members of IPPNW documented and disseminated the health and environmental effects of the production, testing, and use of nuclear weapons. They published research on the tremendous price nuclear armed states are paying in their pursuit of nuclear weaponry in several authoritative books, articles, and op-ed pieces in medical journals. Analysing data on uranium mining, nuclear testing and production, across geographies (from Nevada to Moruroa and Hanford to Chelyabinsk), IPPNW provided the international health community with an assessment of the alarming health and environmental costs of pursuing security through nuclear weapons. Besides raising awareness of these costs, members organised citizens in the nuclear states to protest and influence their governments' policies.

Physician activists were instrumental in the campaigns to ban atmospheric and underground nuclear test explosions and in helping to shut down nuclear weapons testing sites and production facilities. Through the ICAN campaign, which received the 2017 Nobel Peace Prize, they successfully negotiated a treaty on the Prohibition of Nuclear Weapons. Physician members of Medact have also led evidence generation and protests about the harmful effects of **fracking**, and effective campaigns for greener and more sustainable medical practices, food systems, and planet (see Medact's evidence review and risk assessments of fracking available at https://www.medact.org/project/clim ate-health/fracking/).

The UN Conference on Environment and Development held in Rio de Janeiro in 1992 provided a global platform for discussing issues related to economy, environment, and international development. There was unprecedented civil society participation that influenced the official deliberations. By this time, Earth Day, which began on 22 April 1970, had become a popular event across the world, drawing attention to the need for taking action to protect the environment. Global temperatures started rising ominously in the 2000s and some of the hottest ever recorded have occurred since then. The Global Day of Action was launched in 2005 with citizens and civil society organising climate-related rallies and events across the world.

Over the years, civil society organisations, social movements, and individual activists have acted as independent climate watchdogs and activists, participating in conferences as well as protesting and organising direct action. One of the most well-known climate protests was when a 16-year-old school girl from Sweden Greta Thunberg stood outside the Swedish Parliament Riksdag with the sign '*Skolstrejk för klimatet*' or 'School strike for climate' in August 2018. This sparked a series of global strikes in 2019 and inspired the formation of youth climate action groups in several countries, culminating in the UN launching a Youth Advisory Group on Climate Change in 2020. Far away from the strikes in Europe, several women's groups across the world have been taking local action to ensure the environment continues to flourish and nourish the people living there. Along the borders of Syria and Turkey a region that has been devastated by military action, climate change and recently an earthquake, Kurdish women have taken initiatives to bring water for irrigation for their farming cooperatives (Rushton 2023). In India, in the state of Telangana, over 3,000 women have formed collectives to preserve and grow traditional crops like millets, pulses, and greens. These crops are not only more climate resistant but are more nutritious. In Bhuj, a city in the state of Gujarat, people living in low-income settlements, or slums, have taken steps to replenish groundwater, harvest rainwater and clean up lakes to address a growing water shortage (Abraham 2020).

Cases abound on other tactics that activists and advocates have utilised to hold actors accountable to the harms to climate and health. We describe some of these in Chapter 7.

However, change has been slow.

Conclusion: Continuing challenges of politics, economics, and health

Between the time of the Cochabamba Water Wars and COVID-19 pandemic, we can clearly see that the health of populations continues to be affected by a range of global and local political as well as economic factors. During these 20 years there have been many advances in medical technology and the availability of drugs, vaccines, tests, and other medical devices, particularly in the Global South. However, the opportunities for the poor and marginalised to access these advances have also been severely constrained.

One of the defining political features of the post-World War world was the acknowledgement of all individuals being inherently equal as human beings and endowed with the same human rights. Subsequent advances in critical theory helped develop a more nuanced understanding of differences in human condition and lived experiences and how these were influenced by various, social, historical, and economic factors. The field of human rights and public policy has tried to respond to these in several ways (see Chapter 1). The third generation of human rights has constantly been evolving as greater international consensus is obtained on the concerns of disadvantaged groups. New international treaties or conventions related to the rights of women, children, migrants, refugees, persons who are racially discriminated, persons with disabilities, those who are forced into labour, or trafficked have been passed since the International Bill of Human Rights was adopted in 1966. Many countries have made 'inclusive' policies including abolition of apartheid in South Africa, 'affirmative action' in the US, or 'reservation' in India.

The neoliberal economic regimes have supported large corporations with the belief that 'trickle-down' economics will help overall well-being. Instead, over the years there has been rising inequality and impoverishment of the lower income families of the erstwhile socially dominant or privileged populations. In the US, the real wages and standard of living of the working class has hardly increased in the last 40 years (Desilver 2018). Migration due to economic realities or war and conflict into countries of Europe and North America is also creating increased xenophobia. This has led to increased racism and populist politics, evident in movements like Brexit and slogans like Make America Great Again. In India, populist politics is fostering deep divides between the majority Hindu and the minority Muslim population. In academic circles this deterioration of democratic values and processes is variously called democratic back-sliding, de-democratisation, or democratic erosion.

As this chapter illustrated, one of the greatest challenges or barriers to achieve health for all and healthy societies is to tackle the wider political, economic, and environmental determinants of health. Addressing these require interrogating the complex state-market nexus and building accountability of both state and powerful non-state actors. Despite increasing awareness of the health impacts of commercial determinants, and calls by the WHO and other civil society actors to consider the health consequences of their practices, there is still a troubling lack of action by national governments against harmful commercial activities that affect people's health and the planet.

New and complex interactions are emerging out of the neoliberal economic paradigm and populist politics as well as social backlash and ostracism. These affect the health and well-being of marginalised communities but also the way in which public services, including health services, are designed, resourced, delivered, and accessed. As new challenges emerged, new forms of support, mobilisation, and protest have also evolved. The COVID-19 pandemic saw many new forms of social mobilisation, protests, and solidarity to confront the many problems that the pandemic highlighted. These are signs of hope. It must, however, be recognised that we confront a complex political economy. This demands more united resistance that sees struggles for individual claims to justice not in isolation. Links with longstanding historic movements against injustices and alliances with other connected systems in crisis (environment, politics, markets) are crucial to further the agenda of health rights for all.

7

Strengthening accountability for the right to health

Over the past two decades, the notion of accountability of public systems (henceforth referred to as accountability) has gained traction in public and policy debates across several cross-cutting areas of health governance, international aid, and health rights. In this chapter, we provide an overview of theoretical debates on accountability, and provide examples of mechanisms employed by communities to hold duty bearers and other stakeholders to account. Alongside specific examples where community-led accountability mechanisms have been developed and effectively used, we also discuss the limits of such actions in complex unstructured health governance and examine where possibilities for bringing social change lie.

Health policy debates and evaluations often embrace a linear, simplistic, and instrumental understanding of accountability. There is an implied assumption that efficient systems can be achieved simply by enhancing transparency, or making information about system standards and procedures available to citizen groups, providers, and managers. Subsequently through evaluation unsatisfactory or sub-optimal performance can be redressed. On the contrary, the reality of ensuring accountability and operationalising a rights-based approach in public health is far more complex and dynamic. It demands a more holistic understanding of the conditions in which different provider client interactions occur and structural factors and social and political capital that moderate people's engagement. These complexities and challenges in re-distributing power and in negotiating entitlements are highlighted in the chapter through case vignettes of community monitoring processes in select countries.

Introduction to accountability

Broadly speaking, accountability can be understood as the formal and informal processes, norms, and structures, particularly in a democratic system that demands power holders account for their decisions and actions and remedy any failures in delivering their duties (Brinkerhoff 2004; Boydell et al 2018). Attention to accountability has surged in the past decade. This can be attributed in part to the growing international demands for good governance (Cleary, Molyneux, and Gilson 2013), and the much-touted agenda of aid effectiveness pushed at the high-level forums and milestone conferences in Paris and Busan. These initiatives and other landmark conventions and reports (for example, WHO 2019; CSDH 2008) successfully established accountability as a key pathway for improved health and development (Aggarwal and Goodell 2009). It is also considered a core element of improving health systems performance and responsiveness (Brinkerhoff 2003). As a result, the body of research on the role of public and social accountability in bringing about more accessible and better-quality healthcare is growing.

Figure 7.1: Understanding the complexities of accountability

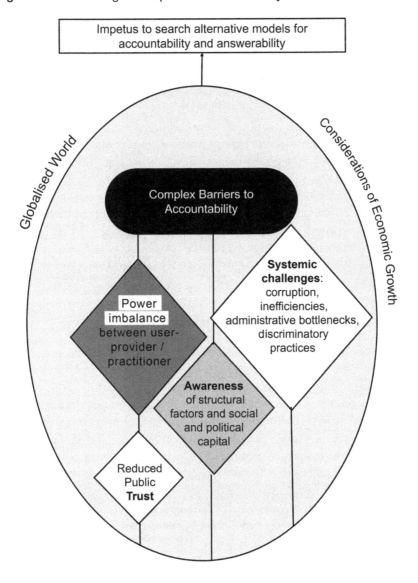

Despite global and national commitments and robust human rights frameworks that guarantee the highest standards of health for all, widening health inequalities and violations of health rights remain a disturbing reality. These have been described in the preceding chapter. Some of the most striking violations take place in sexual and reproductive health services and rights. These are driven, in part, by a growing commercial presence. The high prevalences of unnecessary caesarean section, forced sterilisation, and obstetric violence, especially among vulnerable populations and social minorities are commonplace in healthcare institutions in many countries. Health systems worldwide suffer from poor infrastructure, unavailability of drugs, treatments and qualified healthcare professionals, and unaffordable services. Redressal mechanisms are weak or nonexistent. Even in well-resourced systems of high-income countries, which receive 10 to 17 per cent of GDP allocated to healthcare spending (such as the UK and US), the fragmentation of health and social care systems, decades of underfunding and privatisation worsened by austerity policies have had catastrophic effects on public health systems. These include the health workforce crisis, delayed care, unaffordable treatments, active exclusion of vulnerable populations groups, and gradual erosion of trust in the public health system. These signal an abysmal gap between government obligations and their actual provisions, posing important questions of their answerability to citizens.

We live in a globalised world where decisions on population health are not entirely sovereign; nor are they free from considerations of economic growth. Decision-making power appears diffused amid multiple national and international governance structures, involving both the public and private interests. This makes the practice of accountability both obscure and challenging (see Figure 7.1).

Theoretical overview and historical context

Traditional models of public accountability have been indirect. They involve two interrelated accountability domains: political and bureaucratic. Citizens elect political representatives, granting them authority to govern. If dissatisfied, citizens can withdraw this authority through election. In the bureaucratic process, public bureaucracies assure compliance of procedures in implementing decisions, which are expected to be monitored by elected political representative creating an indirect influence of citizens. This indirect route to accountability not only creates distance between *accountors* and *accountees* (Hupe and Hill 2007) but is affected by several systemic challenges such as corruption, inefficiencies, administrative bottlenecks, and discriminatory practices in public bureaucracies that persist in many countries (McGee and Gaventa 2011; Joshi and Houtzager 2012). At the same time, the failures to deliver services, growing inequities in access to care and rampant violations have resulted in widespread discontent among citizens and civil society and declining trust in the state and public services and institutions.

These failures created an impetus for the search of alternative models or more direct pathways for answerability, often called the short route to accountability. However, the context in which these mechanisms must operate is complex. The rise of public-private partnership (PPP) mode of organisation of health systems involving privately contracted parties to provide functions like finance, provision, as well as regulation blurred the traditional boundaries between state and non-state actors. This created multiple contractual or Principal – Agent (PA) relationships that skew accountability relations (Kapilashrami and Baru 2018). Contemporary health systems include players such as neoliberal markets, civil society, and social movements. These contrasting forces shaped two parallel pathways or streams of accountability that comprise the 'short route' accountability mechanisms (Figure 7.2).

The *first stream*, guided by the New Public Management (NPM) discourse, invokes market mechanisms in the public sector to make managers more accountable and systems more efficient. Joshi and Houtzager (2012) identifies several mechanisms under this. These include both internal mechanisms such as performance-based contracting and financing arrangements, and enhanced incentive environments, as well as external mechanisms such as consumer complaint/grievance redress mechanisms around individual experiences of care. However, studies reveal that these complex chains of delegation are embedded in unequal power relationships and blur responsibilities and accountability relationships (Oliveira Cruz and McPake 2011; Kapilashrami and McPake 2013). Further, their effectiveness is limited in resource-poor contexts by the high levels of distrust in public facilities, attitudes to appeals and fear of counteraction/sanctions from the medical practitioners (McCoy et al 2012), and the exclusion of the poorest and most vulnerable. The *second stream* is concerned with recognising the centrality of rights-based approach and involves participation of citizens in addressing the democratic deficit in governance and decision-making at national and international levels. Health-focused social movements and their activism for health rights are at the heart of these demands and offer a conduit for centring accountability in the health and public policy arena. Their efforts helped formalise the shift from a needs-based to a rights-based approach in providing services and promoting health. Specific actions include the establishment of independent regulatory bodies or authorities such as ombudsperson, and the exercise of the Freedom of Information or the Right to Information acts. These measures hold promise for widening the scope for citizens' forums and civil society to engage more substantively and be more effective watchdogs.

More recently, the discussion has extended to social accountability (Brinkerhoff 2004) or *direct citizen action and engagement*. Distinct from public accountability models that are situated within formal political systems and policy processes, social accountability emphasises sustained and deeper engagement of 'communities', not individuals, to ensure implementation of policy and programmatic provisions. The process through which communities are engaged makes them 'active makers and shapers of services, exercising their rights as citizens' (Cornwall 2000). Joshi and Houtzager (2012) refer to *participatory democracy* wherein citizens directly engage with different levels of bureaucracies and policy processes through local governance and village assemblies to mainstream rights–based approaches in service provision (Cornwall and Coelho 2007). Here, organising and capacitating vulnerable groups to confront disempowering relations and develop strategies for addressing causes of neglect can ultimately transform relationships between the dominant elite and the oppressed.

Figure 7.2: Formal and informal accountability mechanisms

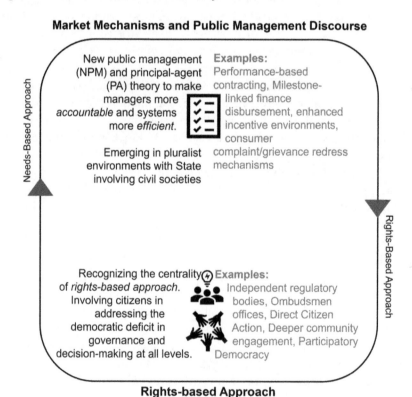

Market Mechanisms and Public Management Discourse

New public management (NPM) and principal-agent (PA) theory to make managers more accountable and systems more *efficient*.

Examples: Performance-based contracting, Milestone-linked finance disbursement, enhanced incentive environments, consumer complaint/grievance redress mechanisms

Emerging in pluralist environments with State involving civil societies

Recognizing the centrality of *rights-based approach*. Involving citizens in addressing the democratic deficit in governance and decision-making at all levels.

Examples: Independent regulatory bodies, Ombudsmen offices, Direct Citizen Action, Deeper community engagement, Participatory Democracy

Needs-Based Approach

Rights-Based Approach

Rights-based Approach

In a nutshell, social accountability can be understood as continuing engagement of citizens and civil society and their collective actions to hold states to account and ensure provision of quality public goods. Support from donors, civil societies, and some national governments has resulted in social accountability gaining traction for health system reforms and improvements (Hoffmann 2014). Citizen-led or community-based accountability initiatives took development by storm in the early 2000s, independently or as part of community development projects, in health. These initiatives are usually led by community members who are trained by NGOs to undertake various tasks at a health facility or community level. Some examples include citizens monitoring of public services, community audits of health outcomes (for example, for maternal deaths and obstetric care), and participatory gender budgeting. As these accountability initiatives grew in scale and geographic scope, there was growing interest in understanding and evaluating their effectiveness. One such initiative is that of the Community-based Monitoring that was introduced in the National Rural Health Mission by the Government of India in 2008, in partnership with the civil society. It is briefly described next.

Case study 7.1: Community-based monitoring and planning in India

The Community-based Monitoring and Planning (CBMP) initiative was implemented in 2008 as a partnership between the Government of India and civil society organisations. It was a result of longstanding engagement of activists (members of the People's Health Movement) in health advocacy with the state that culminated in the development of a community-based monitoring approach within the framework of the National Rural Health Mission (NRHM) (GOI 2005). 'Communitisation' was seen as key to facilitate the processes of demand-side accountability and the formation of Village-level Health and Sanitation Committees (VHSC) to institutionalise such mechanisms in the healthcare system. The geographic scope covered 324 primary health centres (PHCs) in 36 districts in nine states in India. The initiative was developed as an accountability and oversight mechanism for effective functioning of primary healthcare, and to increase community's awareness, negotiating space and power to seek their entitlements within the health systems. It was operationalised in the health systems through the formation of VHSC, a representative body comprising health service providers at the community level, elected representatives from local governance institutions, CSOs, and members of the community. These VHSCs were responsible for planning services appropriate to health needs of the community and to ensure continued monitoring of guaranteed health services with meaningful participation of all constituent members. Citizens' interaction with the various levels of health system was enabled via distinct phases of action involving:

1. community organising and awareness raising of healthcare entitlements;
2. capacity building of VHSC members and other key community leaders, with a focus on the contents of the NRHM and tools and processes of evaluating health services;

3. evidence collection on status and performance of health services via surveys, interviews, and in-depth case studies and its synthesis into report cards. The cards indicated the level of functioning of the health system coded in traffic signal colours (for example, red implied defunct services, yellow suggested sub-optimal performance and green for well-functioning system);

4. public dialogues (jan samwads) that served as a platform for citizens to share findings from facility appraisals and engage health providers and facility officials at different levels viz. PHC, community health centre, district, and state.

These phases were not run as discrete activities but as an iterative process of evidence generation, dialogue, and monitoring for corrective action and improvement in the system.

Reviews and independent evaluation of the process showed improvements in the community's awareness of health issues and entitled services as well as changes in the health service quality and access, achieved through local mobilisation and use of locally produced informative material. Most notable, however, was a strengthened public discourse on democratisation of health and accountability. Spaces created as part of the CBMP process continued to leverage dialogue between community members and healthcare providers, in the process empowering communities to seek prompt action from providers and local governance (for example, Panchayat Raj Institution (PRI) members) in case of emergencies. By linking local awareness of entitlements and actual state of services to the accountability chain of higher authorities in the health system through regular feedback loops, communities were able to draw attention to (and improve) a range of other public services and determinants of health. For example, filling up vacancies of sanitation workers, reinstating patient welfare committees, and attention to a range of local healthcare demands in the official plan (for example, introducing treatment of diabetes and hypertension, changes in hygiene in PHCs and subcentres). (Sources: SATHI 2010; Khanna and Pradhan 2013; Shukla, Saha, and Jadhav 2013)

Operationalising accountability

Citizens and civil societies have adopted a range of actions, strategies, and instruments to operationalise accountability in health systems and promote answerability of health policy makers, managers, and providers. These include:

• Establishing structures such as community-led forums and village-level health committees (as described in case study 7.1) that are responsible for monitoring and planning services;

• Specific mechanisms and processes to improve services and facilities (for example, community audits through which citizens participated in monitoring and improving service provision, and budgeting);

- Advocating for reforms in health legislation, policies, programmes, and budgetary allocations for furthering accountability.

Health manifestos or service charters have served as effective tools for such advocacy efforts to lobby political parties and public authorities at national and sub-national levels.

Health service charters (for example, in Kenya) are jointly drafted by patients and providers, through participatory processes, to list the available services at a health facility, along with information on costs, waiting times, and facility hours, providing the baseline for citizens to assess the services they receive and hold providers accountable.

Health manifestos on the other hand are bold statements of collective vision and demands generated through a participatory process informed by people's lived experiences. We describe this process in Chapter 5, in the context of organising for health rights in Scotland (see the image of the PHM Manifesto in Figure 7.3).

Social accountability mechanisms such as those described before provide citizens' direct access to negotiate with public authorities using their own

Figure 7.3: People's Health Manifesto for Scotland

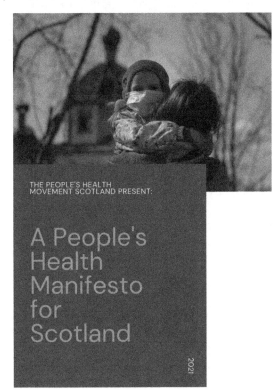

experiences as key evidence. However, their effective implementation and uptake is contingent on the creation of enabling dialogic spaces conducive for effective governance. To support these, social movements have used national legislation (for example, freedom of information or right to information act) to invoke transparency and accountability through legal means, and international human rights instruments and agreements adopted at specific conventions to monitor states' progress. Some of these are outlined as follows.

Box 7.1: Examples of legislation to formalise community participation in accountability initiatives

Annual public hearings and civil society representation on the decision-making board for essential health services in *Thailand* stem from provisions in the Universal Health Coverage legislation (the National Health Security Act) that provide for inclusion of the voice and concerns of citizens (Kantamaturapoj et al 2020).

In *Brazil* social participation is a guiding principle for the Unified Health System enshrined in the country's constitution and in law, including specifically in legislation pertaining to health technology assessments and decision-making (Silva et al 2019).

In *India*, 'communitisation' became a core element of the National Rural Health Mission in India, enabling the formation and implementation of village health committees and community-based monitoring initiative, and legitimising actions to hold duty bearers to account for health rights violation (Dasgupta 2011).

A formal international mechanism exists through the Human Rights Council (HRC). Established in 2006, the HRC promotes 'universal respect for the protection of all human rights and fundamental freedoms for all, without distinction of any kind'. It has established the mechanism of the Universal Periodic Review that uses 'objective and reliable information, of the fulfilment by each state of its human rights obligations and commitments'. The HRC also introduced Special Rapporteurs, who were independent human rights experts to report and advise the HRC on thematic and country-specific issues. These mechanisms have allowed activists, social movements, and other civil society organisations, both at the country level and internationally, opportunities to provide direct feedback and counterpoints to country-level submissions on their human rights obligations. The counterpoint report provided by civil societies to the official country-level reports to UN Treaty bodies like the *Committee on the Elimination of Discrimination against Women* (CEDAW), *International Covenant on Civil and Political Rights* (ICCPR), and *International Covenant on Economic, Social and Cultural Rights* (ICESCR) are referred to as 'Shadow Reports', and these are used by these treaty bodies in preparing their concluding observations.

The Special Rapporteur on the Right to Health has prepared many issue-focused thematic reports with extensive inputs from civil society, and via country-level visits to countries like Peru, Uganda, Mozambique, India, Australia, Malaysia, and others. Some prominent thematic reports were on HIV/AIDS, Access to Medicines, Bioethics, Mental Health, Maternal health among others. These reports are tabled at the Human Rights Council and are available on the website of the Special Rapporteur on the Right to Health of the Office of the High Commissioner on Human Rights.

Courts at the national and international courts like the InterAmerican Court and the European Court of Human Rights have also been used by social movements for health-related human rights violations. One such country case involving Healthwatch petitioning in the Supreme Court is presented in Chapter 8.

In a nutshell, contrary to the linear and mechanism-based understanding of accountability, an 'ecosystem' of accountability exists. An 'accountability ecosystem' (Van Belle et al 2018) constitutes a range of actors, with diverse roles, responsibilities, and interactions – from global to the local – and accountability strategies that are linked, not mutually exclusive. However, this ecosystem remains insufficiently utilised in health policy and systems, and not uniformly developed or resourced in most countries.

'Accountability ecosystem': community organising for systems reform

The case study of community-based monitoring and planning (CBMP) in India reveals the 'accountability ecosystem' that utilises several linked mechanisms and strategies. These are identified in Figures 7.4 and 7.5.

The impact associated with community-based monitoring must however be historically situated and understood in the context of wider social movements from which these accountability strategies emerged and which in turn strengthened these movements. For example, the establishment of the CBMP initiative resulted from the health rights activism that followed the establishment of the people's health movement in 2000 (described in Chapter 6 on Social Movements). However, the momentum around it can be traced back to the experiences of the health rights mobilisation and grassroots struggles of the 1970s and 1980s, such as environmental movements protesting deforestation and construction of large dams that displaced rural poor and affected their lives and livelihoods. Similarly, in health space, sustained campaigns (supported by participatory approaches and action research introduced in Chapter 9) and health-related rights mobilisation that took place in the preceding decades created fertile grounds for the success of the initiative. These campaigns targeted the coercive population policy and the two-child norm, coercive promotion of hazardous long-acting contraceptive technologies that were being pushed through donor-driven family planning programmes and targeted approach; issues that supported organising for women's reproductive health rights.

The historical backdrop helps us appreciate the context in which theory and praxis of social accountability evolved and gained currency. The concerted effort of various actors that paved way for uptake of such radical policy propositions is not simply a precursor but a precondition for subsequent reforms and must be considered when discussing scalability of accountability initiatives. For example, people's organisations active in Maharashtra played a key role in refining the monitoring tool and ensuring participation of people beyond the pilot phase financed by the government (Khanna and Pradhan 2013).

Capacity building, evidence gathering, and public dialogues were not discrete activities but integral to the processes of empowering and organising communities to assert their democratic power to question and demand accountability from the authorities and for continuously negotiating changes in the healthcare system. Even within this, while professional NGOs prioritised the technicality of formation of VHSCs, training communities on assessing services, the people's organisations prioritised community action and citizens' participation for accountability (SATHI 2010).

The public hearings became an effective tool for promoting accountability of the system by providing a platform to citizens from 30 states for presenting grievances and complaints along with solutions from the communities. Neera Chandhoke (2007), in her analysis of the public hearing, highlights three functions that help deepen democracy: (1) producing informed citizens; (2) encouraging citizens to participate in local affairs through the provision of information and social auditing; and (3) creating a sense of civic responsibility by bringing people together to address issues of collective concern. The CBMP process, especially the component of public hearings, therefore helped leverage democratic participation of the citizens in health accountability and health planning besides democratising the health system by holding officials accountable and answerable to citizens.

Walter Flores and members of the Community of Practitioners on Accountability and Social Action in Health (COPASAH) initiative draw on several years of community organising, advocacy experience, and literature to highlight key pre-conditions for effective interventions that strengthen citizens' voice and system reforms. These, as illustrated in Figure 7.4, include:

- Provisions for accessing and disseminating information regarding health system priorities, entitlements, and programme provisions and service delivery.
- Organising communities around the need for health services and entitlements as well as building community capacity for monitoring services. NGOs play a key role in these two aspects.

- A trustworthy and accessible system for grievance redressal which is mandated and operated by the state authorities.
- Institutionalisation of corrective action for sustained improvement and revised priority setting.

These pre-conditions highlight the importance of amplifying voices at the community level, while also emphasising the need for a 'compact' that supports system reforms at institutional level. This compact focuses on utilising state-centric mechanisms and creating incentive structures that promote accountability among providers and power holders.

These pre-conditions are integrated and expanded as 'core principles' for meaningful community engagement within the Assessing Community Engagement (ACE) conceptual model. The model situates community engagement as core to achieving and accelerating progress toward the goal of health equity through strengthened health systems. The four 'propellers' emanate from this core, reflecting major domains and outcomes of engaging communities. Impact in these domains leads to the fundamental goal of health equity and systems transformation and is contextualised by the drivers of health; drivers of change; and the social, political, racial, economic, historical, and environmental context. Together, the ACE model and the previously identified pre-conditions provide insight into the diverse and intricate accountability ecosystem required for driving change.

Critical gaps on social accountability

The role of accountability is well established in the health policy and systems field. It has ranged from closing the democratic deficit in global health governance (by watching and targeting conflict of interests, calling for greater transparency and accountability) to reforming national health systems and local planning processes in the struggle to achieve health for all. Studies on social accountability mechanisms highlight improvements in governance, service delivery, quality of care and health outcomes, empowerment of citizens, and reforms in health and other public systems (George et al 2015; Boydell et al 2019). Besides these tangible outcomes, community-led accountability initiatives serve as useful learning sites for participants to become more aware of local services and other community assets and their functioning and provide unique information and experiential knowledge that remain peripheral to health planning and policy narratives (D'Ambruoso et al 2013; Samuel, Flores, and Frisancho 2020). These are critical to create the empowered communities that can facilitate change.

Despite consensus on these benefits, doubts are cast over the dearth of evidence on their effectiveness, methodological challenges around measuring their impact, and the failure to account for confounding interventions and

Figure 7.4: Pre-conditions for success of strengthening citizens' voice

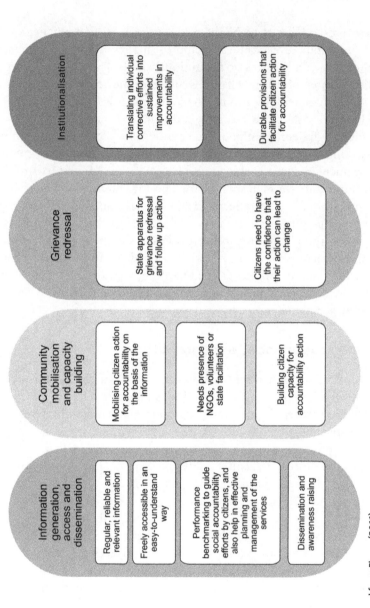

Source: Reproduced from Flores (2011)

Figure 7.5: Core principles and domains of change in Assessing Community Engagement (ACE) (adapted and re-drawn)

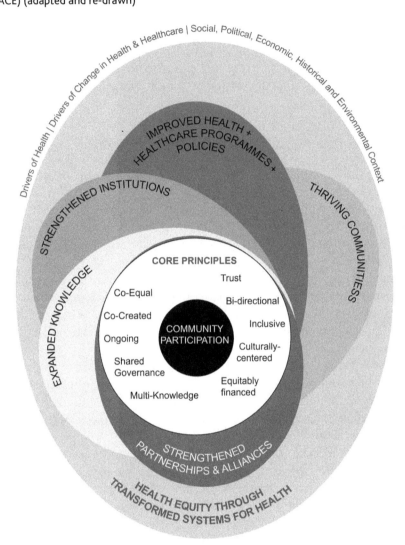

Source: Adaptation of 'Assessing Community Engagement (ACE) Conceptual Model' from National Academy of Medicine (n.d.)

health system factors that may influence outcomes such as quality of care (McCoy et al 2012; Molyneux et al 2012).

Notably, *three key conceptual gaps/challenges* limit possibilities for studying and transferring lessons to improve accountability practice.

The first concerns the ambiguity in their scope and diversity in purposes. Social accountability initiatives can take different forms based on the distinct objectives they serve. These can include effective citizens' engagement in decision-making and monitoring the exercise of public authority (Peruzzotti et al 2006) or tracking progress and performance leading to service reforms and fostering empowerment (Papp, Gogoi, and Campbell 2013). Differences may also arise based on what triggers accountability initiatives. Triggers could be demand-side pressures from users/communities or supply-side reforms. For instance, Joshi and Houtzager (2012) argue that methodological choices to assess accountability initiatives, and change efforts and reforms more broadly, are made in the context of donor-enforced impact assessment designs and top-down monitoring and evaluation frameworks that further marginalise poor and vulnerable populations the systems are meant to serve. Differences can also be due to the different contexts in which these emerge, the assumptions they are premised on, and the theory of change that underpins them.

Casting such differences in the motives and ideologies that drive distinct accountability mechanisms as mainly methodological and technical obscures the fundamental issues 'which are about power and politics, not methodological technicalities' (McGee and Gaventa 2011, p 3). This conceptual distinction, Joshi and Houtzager (2012) argue, is significant as it determines the yardstick on which accountability mechanisms are assessed.

A related second problem is the discursive understanding of accountability that is dominant in mainstream policy narrative. Here, accountability is viewed as a linear and simplistic process through which system reforms and efficiency in social sector spending can be achieved by a two-stage process. This involves, at first, enhancing transparency to ensure information is available in the public domain and accessible to citizen groups, providers, and managers in health facilities. Right to information (RTI) or freedom of information (FOI) mechanisms are usually adopted for this purpose. This is then followed by initiatives to evaluate services for appropriateness and quality of care and correct unsatisfactory or sub-standard performance. Such linear conceptualisation overlooks the hierarchical and complex nature of health systems and power dynamics in which provider-citizen/client relationships and transactions are embedded. It also ignores the deep inequalities and social exclusion that prevent certain population groups from accessing available information or exercising their rights and exposes the limits of adopting an empirical approach to community health.

The reality of ensuring responsive health systems and operationalising a rights-based approach in health is more complex. It involves a better understanding of the conditions in which negotiations occur and how people's engagement is moderated by structural factors and social and political capital (McGee and Gaventa 2011; Gaventa and McGee 2013). Yet, the initiatives tend to be presented rather statically, studied cross-sectionally, with limited attention to the wider conditions under which their distinct objectives are met. We therefore stress a dynamic view of accountability that must examine the multiple – distinct and overlapping – pathways to change, and key contextual elements which determine these.

A third gap relates to the deeply contested nature and articulation of mainstreaming community/citizen's participation, a crucial element in the accountability process. The mainstreaming of accountability has received much criticism. These include running the risk of increasing co-option and instrumentalisation, its incompatibility with top-down planning systems in which institutional practices of development are embedded as well as the lack of attention to political processes and power in generating evidence on their effectiveness (Cooke and Kothari 2001; Mosse 2001; Kapilashrami and O'Brien 2012).

Assessment of community participation in accountability initiatives appears strikingly cautious. Concerns are many. One such concern is around tokenism in composition of committees and their mandates and whether there is true devolution of power and democratic functioning. Another is the lack of awareness and inadequate capacities of both community members, as well as authorities in managing participatory governance processes (Boydell et al 2019; Arthur, Saha, and Kapilashrami 2023). Several studies have highlighted how accountability initiatives tend to scratch the surface and seldom tackle the structural and systemic causes. The issues often ignored include underfunding and austerity measures, mismanagement, corruption, and neglect as well as entrenched inequalities and social exclusion that continue to plague health systems, and in the community engagement in planning, in most parts of the world (Samuel, Flores, and Frisancho 2020; Flores and Samuel 2019).

Corporate accountability and citizens action

A black hole in accountability scholarship concerns the actions and conflicting interests of corporations and the commercial sector. While an increasing proportion of global burden of diseases is attributable to what is commonly referred to as 'lifestyle' diseases and 'behavioural' risk factors, there is mounting evidence that the underlying aetiology is overconsumption of unhealthy products (tobacco, food and drinks high in fat, salt and sugar, alcohol, and other substances) that are produced and aggressively promoted by commercial entities. As described in Chapter 6, the corporate influence in health goes beyond supplying and marketing these products (Dorfman et al 2012). There is growing evidence and concern about the commercial sector's influence in health policy. The commercial sector and its practices influence health in several ways. They influence policy agendas (Collin et al 2017), and frame health problems and solutions in a reductive and primarily clinical approach. For example, reducing it to individual biomedical factors and away from its social determinants or upstream drivers. They adopt a range of tactics to limit the role of the state in regulating harmful practices (Lima and Galea 2018). Corporations resist statutory regulation, promote self-regulation via voluntary codes, and coopt the language of participatory citizenship in Corporate Social Responsibility (CSR) initiatives. Entitlement claims made in these initiatives are seldom accompanied with assuming obligations (Newell 2006).

Further, private healthcare accounts for a substantial proportion of healthcare spending in several nations (as high as 70 to 80 per cent in select countries). This sector is highly heterogenous, comprising large corporate hospitals, smaller nursing homes, and clinics of individual practitioners. Medical practice in these settings remains largely unregulated and characterised by insidious links between drug companies and their representatives, travel agencies promoting medical tourism, unscrupulous practices to increase profits (for example, for unnecessary procedures and surgeries), and weak laws and monitoring practices that regulate this sector (Kapilashrami et al 2016). Furthermore, the growing trend of private equity and financialisation of healthcare has meant a greater presence of large corporations in setting up health infrastructure and financing (Hamer and Kapilashrami 2020).

In view of these developments, several critical questions emerge. How can traditional or contemporary modes of accountability be extended beyond the state to hold the commercial sector to account for their harmful practices? How can the dangers associated with co-optation, aggressive marketing, and insidious practices of the corporate sector be mitigated and corporate injustices effectively countered?

Over the years, activists and social movements (including organisations such as Health Action International, Medact, International Physicians for the Prevention of Nuclear War (IPPNW), People's Health Movement (PHM) among others) have adopted several strategies to call out these injustices and hold actors to account. While these are further detailed in Chapter 6, broadly these include: (1) documenting evidence and assessing the impact of industry practices and activities on lives, livelihoods, and health (for example, the Union Carbide gas leak, the impact of fracking on health), (2) challenging the ways in which social and environmental impact assessments are made, (3) demanding compensation for lost lives and disability, and (4) promoting shareholder activism and strategies such as disrupting annual general meetings and lobbying. A further action domain, one that is advanced by the health movements, is to influence the terms of engagement with corporations at the national or global level. An example of this is the advocacy for the FENSA process to inform WHO's engagement with non-state and commercial actors. However, the impact of citizens' action in this sphere, and corporate responsiveness, remains limited in the absence of an effective welfare-oriented pro-poor state.

Conclusion: Engendering future agenda for accountable systems and societies

Enriching theory and praxis on accountability demand an expansion of the field in multiple domains. Empirically, more research, particularly ontologically diverse research, is needed to understand content (that is, the design of initiatives and mechanism), process (how they are working), overarching context (socio-political and institutional factors), and the underlying conditions that make these strategies and practices responsive, equitable and effective for all, specifically for the socially excluded and marginalised.

Conceptually, the field needs to expand to investigate strategies and effects, not only in the specific context of improving public health services (and making them more responsive) but also for democratising the unstructured and diffused governance at national, regional, and global levels. This requires extending and branching out enquiry into the corporate-state nexus and the global-local assemblages in which contemporary health systems operate. Accountability initiatives and efforts to achieve health equity and rights must also reflect the evolving notions of community's role and participation: from passive beneficiaries, and tokenistic representation to active empowered citizens.

PART III

Tools for transformation and organising for change: arts, media, and participatory action research

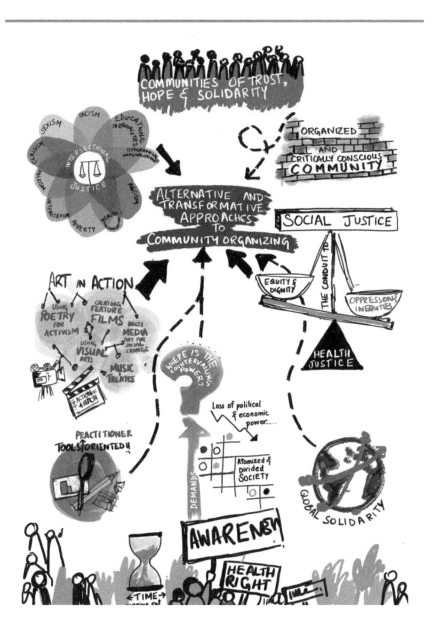

8

Community activism in action

The COVID-19 pandemic was probably the most significant health event globally in recent years. There have been several health scares since the beginning of the new millennium like SARS, Swine flu, Ebola and Zika, but COVID-19 was by far the most devastating. Between 2020 to 2022, the pandemic came back in waves and by the time it was under some form of control over 700 million people across 229 countries had been infected and over 7 million had died. When the pandemic was announced in March 2020, countries across the world announced restrictions on movement. On the one hand, individuals and communities were confused, frightened, or desperate from the mixed messages received from diverse sources, triggering global panic and considerable unrest everywhere. But on the other hand, communities and civil society organisations also took many initiatives to reach out to those in distress. Pandemics provide an interesting window to understand the nature of community activism. In this chapter we will explore the nature and possibilities of community activism for furthering better health and health rights for all using several examples. The central thesis of this chapter is that advocacy and activism are essential components of public health's efforts to achieve health rights and greater health equity. Community activism and social movements serve as critical conduits and a decisive force in this struggle for healthier societies and a fairer world.

The COVID-19 pandemic: State response and community activism

India provides an interesting case study to understand community activism during the COVID-19 pandemic. The first case of COVID-19 was reported from India towards the end of January 2020. A month later India hosted a state visit by the US President Donald Trump. At that time the spread of the infection was slow, and the death rates were miniscule compared to what was being reported from countries in Europe. On 11 March 2020, WHO declared COVID-19 to be a pandemic. India continued with health advisories and cursory testing. On 22 March the Prime Minister urged the people of the country to observe 'voluntary curfew' from dawn to dusk and felicitate health workers engaged in COVID-19-related duties by banging utensils at a specific hour (PIB 2020). The very next day the Government of India announced a national 'lockdown' starting 24 hours later. All movement and economic activities came to a standstill. The short notice period meant there was very little time for preparation, and people were stuck in their homes without food or even water because millions lacked piped water.

Many civil society organisations, businesses, and volunteers swung into action, coordinating over their mobile phones, arranging cooked meals, dry rations, and sanitisers and protective equipment. Soon there was a swelling stream of migration as the informal workers from urban centres started moving back to their villages. It is estimated that nearly 60 million people moved back to their homes during 2020. Initially there was very little support extended by the government. During this phase, civil society groups reached out to help the migrants in many ways. Kitchens were set up on the migrants' routes; they were even provided with footwear. When transport arrangements started, volunteers helped to identify available routes and transportation and coordinate with the authorities. Several social media groups were formed for coordination and portals set up to collect donations. When the second wave of COVID-19 hit the country in early 2021 the health system was overwhelmed. Hospital beds and even oxygen cylinders were unavailable even in the big cities (including the national capital). Various formal and informal groups stepped in provide a range of support as public and private healthcare systems floundered (Siyech and Jouhar 2020; Duvendack and Sonne 2021; Misra 2021; Tandon and Aravind 2021; Sapra and Nayak 2021).

In addition to the restrictions imposed by lockdowns, states also used violence against civilians to enforce these. Excessive use of force to maintain these lockdown restrictions were reported from all over the world. A global report on conflicts and demonstrations noted that in the first year of the pandemic, state repression increased around the world (ACLED 2021). In India, migrants who were fleeing cities to return home were beaten with batons, sprayed with bleaching powder, and compelled to walk hundreds of kilometres (NCAT 2020; Rashid 2020; Biswas 2020). In Uganda, 12 persons were killed by security forces to enforce COVID-19 restrictions when the country confirmed its first COVID-19 case (BBC News 2020). In Nigeria, the Director of Amnesty International's country office noted 'we are also concerned by reports and videos circulating on social media showing violations of human rights, that include beatings by law enforcement agencies tasked with ensuring compliance with the lockdown' (Amnesty International 2020).

Soon after lockdowns were introduced, Clement Voule, the UN Special Rapporteur on the Rights to Freedom of Peaceful Assembly and of Association, issued a statement drawing attention to a 'militarisation of crisis management'. While saluting governments for taking necessary measures, he asked them to be cautious about using measures 'geared more at cementing control and cracking down on oppositional figures than at ensuring public health' (OHCHR 2020). He advised that states should consider civil society as an essential partner and involve them in several roles including framing inclusive policies and providing support to vulnerable populations. Unfortunately, the restrictions were often selective, and their impact most strongly felt by marginalised groups. In the city of New York, one of the more severely affected cities at that time, Latino and Black people were twice as likely to die than white people, and the infection was concentrated in those ZIP codes where poorer people lived (Wade 2020). These measures also disproportionately affected migrants, women from ethnic minorities and refugees and those in institutionalised settings like prisons, detention centres and camps in Europe (Germain and Yong 2020; Hankivsky and Kapilashrami 2020).

In Europe after the first wave of COVID-19 had subsided, street protests broke out in several cities as the Delta wave started spreading. Brussels saw tens of thousands of people marching on the streets, opposing COVID-19 passes. In The Hague, protestors set bicycles on fire. In Vienna, 40,000 people marched protesting against lockdown and compulsory vaccination (Reuters 2021). In Paris, Hamburg, Prague, Luxemburg, and many other cities, hundreds and sometimes thousands of people were on the streets protesting the new restrictions that were imposed because of the emerging Delta wave of the pandemic) (BBC 2021; Aljazeera 2022; DW 2022). Such widespread protests were unprecedented.

A CIVICUS report (2021) noted that in over 100 countries protestors were detained for failure to abide by COVID-19 related guidelines. There were reports of the use of excessive force by security forces from 79 countries and protestors were reported killed in at least 28 countries. There were protests in 59 countries for what was classified as anti-confinement measures or various kinds of restrictions like quarantine, curfew and lockdowns. In 42 countries there were protests for labour and sector demands which included protests by doctors and other healthcare workers demanding better protective equipment or work conditions. Workers from different sectors like hospitality, manufacturing, construction, and others protested asking for financial support, workplace protection, or against inhumane working conditions, or lack of work. There were protests around food insecurity, poverty, unemployment, and similar issues which the report terms as economic, social, and cultural rights in at least 33 countries. Protests demanding better conditions for migrants, refugees, or prisoners also took place in many countries (see Figure 8.1).

Human rights in times of pandemics: a brief history

Pandemics have been historically associated with sequestering of people and goods and restrictions on movement. Protests associated with the HIV/AIDS

Figure 8.1: State and public reactions and responses to public health emergencies

Facilitative Policy Measures   **Support**

-Siracusa Principles   Information Dissemination-
-Relief measures for most   Volunteering-
affected population groups   Support Groups-
-Addressing inequalities,   Community Catering-
-Trust & Collaboration   Coalitions-
-Faster & Agile Responses

| Government | Public Health Emergencies | Communities |

-Compulsory Vaccination   Violent Protests-
-Confinement measures   Shooting/ Firing-
-Riot Police   Street Protests-
-Militarised crisis Management   State Distrust-
-Authoritarian Regimes   Mob/ Riots-
-Democratic Deficit   Resisting health safety measures-

Coercive Policy Measures &   **Protests**
Authoritarian Actions

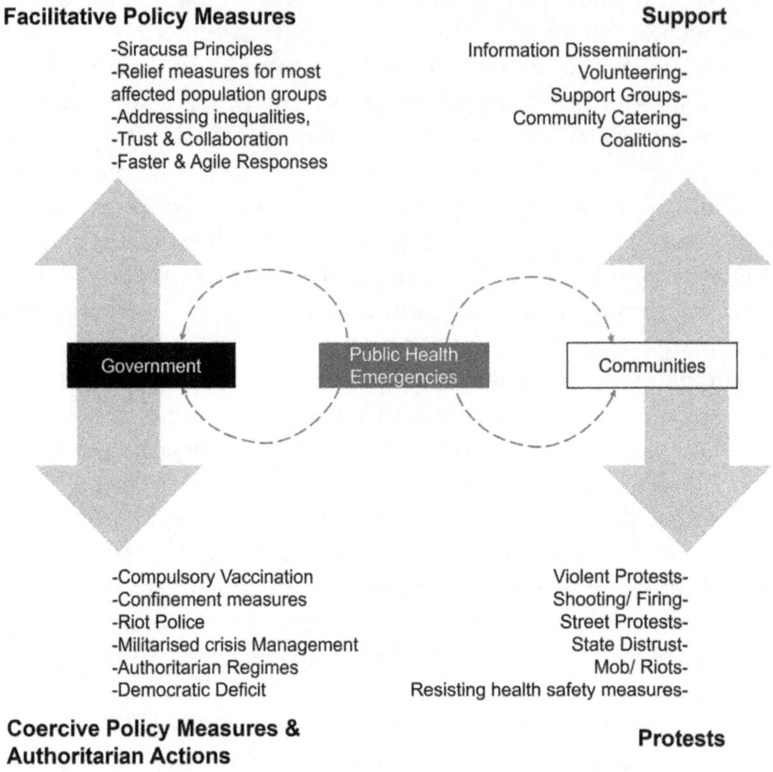

pandemic have been referred to in earlier chapters (see Chapters 2 and 4). Quarantine (from the Italian word *quaranta* or 40) was introduced during the Black Death (plague) pandemic of the fourteenth century. At that time, it was thought that plague spread through the 'pestilential air' and ships, which were suspected to have infected sailors or passengers, were isolated, fumigated, and held for 40 days at quarantine stations. Starting with Italian cities, this practice then spread to the rest of Europe (Tognotti 2013).

Quarantine and isolation emerged as common practice to prevent the spread of plague and were then used against other epidemics like yellow fever, cholera, influenza, and even polio and Ebola in the eighteenth, nineteenth, twentieth, and even twenty-first century. Although a cornerstone of organised national and international response to disease outbreaks for centuries, these practices have been controversial for their political, ethical, and rights implications. Forcefully moving infected people away, as well as myths and misconceptions about the disease, have also led to protests and riots during pandemics over the centuries. Plague riots took place in Moscow in 1771. As the disease spread in the city of Moscow, the rich went off to the countryside and the poor were shut out from their homes and pushed to the streets, and contaminated buildings were burnt down. Confused and angry, the poor rioted and broke into the Kremlin (Pearce 2020). Widespread riots also took place in several places in Europe during the cholera epidemic in 1830s. A conspiracy theory gained ground that the disease was being spread by the government, doctors, and other elites to kill the poor (Johnson 2020).

However, community activism during the COVID-19 pandemic was not only through protests. Mention has already been made of how in India communities stepped in to support people in distress. A review of civil society and citizen response to the COVID-19 pandemic based on 200 case studies of diverse kinds of organisations from various countries found three key patterns in the nature of the support that they were able to provide. First, these groups were able to use digital technology in different ways. This included providing information and services to mobilising resources to organising for protests and advocacy. The review also found that these organisations were able to provide a 'faster and more agile response'. During the pandemic CSOs were also able to facilitate coalition-building, often blurring the lines between formal and informal civil society. CSOs were able to function even though they were faced with authoritarian regimes and restrictions in several places (Nampoothiri and Artuso 2021).

Pandemics, public health and human rights

The balance between public good and individual freedoms has been a classic dilemma within the 'right to health' approach and management of epidemics and pandemics provide a very good example. According to Article 29 of the Universal Declaration of Human Rights (UDHR) which deals with rights with respect to the community, rights may be checked only where such limitations 'are determined by law solely for the purpose of securing due recognition and respect for the rights and freedoms of others and of meeting the just requirements of morality, public order and the general welfare in a democratic society'. Considering the long history of coercive public health measures some experts have advised 'it may be useful to adopt the maxim that health policies and programmes should be considered discriminatory and burdensome on human rights until proven otherwise' (Mann et al 1994).

The Siracusa Principles (illustrated in Figure 8.2) provide guidance on how states can balance between necessary restrictions and rights during emergencies including in public health emergencies like the COVID-19 pandemic. These principles were articulated by a group of experts in 1984 to prevent governments from arbitrarily repressing and denying the rights of individuals in the name of national or public interest and delineated conditions and circumstances by which rights laid down in the ICCPR may be limited or 'derogated'. The Siracusa Principles advise these conditions must be strictly necessary, the least intrusive or restrictive, guided by evidence, non-discriminatory and limited in their application, and subject to review (UNECOSOC 1984). The Siracusa Principles were accepted by the UN Economic and Social Council (ECOSOC) but their non-binding nature limit their enforceability.

A review of various public policy measures to manage pandemics and epidemics, including the latest COVID-19 pandemic, indicate that states all over the world and at different points in the pandemic have probably resorted to measures which could be construed as oppressive by many people. And people have protested. Human rights advisories are consistent in their recommendation that public policies and measures, including those in such crises, need to be inclusive, participatory, transparent, and accountable. However, experience indicates that they are seldom so. There are confusions, misinformation, opaque decision-making processes, and the poor and marginalised communities are more often than not disproportionately affected and have protested.

Figure 8.2: Siracusa principles

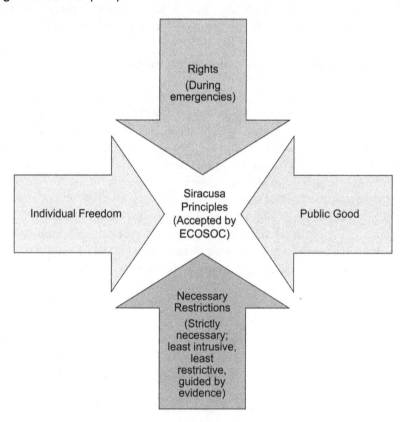

Advocacy: a different form of civil society activism

Advocacy has emerged as a popular and officially endorsed mechanism for civil society activism for policy change at the local, national, and global levels. Unlike civil society activism that often emerges in a more spontaneous manner, advocacy is more deliberate and planned. Advocacy is usually aimed at persuading official bodies to change their actions and policies. It draws its legitimacy from local, national, or global legal or policy standards. Any robust advocacy needs to derive its strength from the experiences and energy of the community. But since advocacy at its core includes a negotiation for change with public authorities, it often uses formal mechanisms, expert intermediaries and formal platforms. Described next is a two-decade-long advocacy experience around coercive population policies and family planning in India.

Advocacy against coercive population policies and for reproductive health and rights in India

Setting the context – India is now the most populous country in the world and population growth has been a key policy concern since independence. Population control is considered key to the alleviation of poverty and development in public policy. In 1966 a separate Department of Family Planning was established within the Ministry of Health to tackle the problem. In the early 1970s mega-sterilisation camps, mostly for men, became popular. In 1975 the then Prime Minister, Indira Gandhi, declared an 'Emergency' and all civil political rights were suspended. During the 18 months of emergency, millions of vasectomy operations were conducted, often forcefully in such camps (Connelly 2006).

After the emergency the family planning programme was renamed Family Welfare but soon became coercive again. The programmatic focus had now shifted and women's sterilisation or tubectomy was now aggressively pursued through incentives and targets (Anil 1994). Officials from the village level upwards coaxed, cajoled, and coerced women to adopt family planning methods, and surgeons boasted how deftly and quickly they could conduct tubal ligation in minutes (Dhanraj 1991). The poor experienced family planning as a compulsion to undergo sterilisation operations, if they were to access any government benefits.

Population Control also manifested itself also through the two-child policy introduced in the early 1990s. The two-child policy compelled families to limit their family size in order to receive public services and appointments. Women were adversely impacted with the introduction of the two-child norm (Visaria, Acharya, and Raj 2006). Since the norm was applied for couples who would have a third child after the norm was announced (in the future) younger women were the worst affected. Further, due to son-preference and gender discriminatory attitudes in society, the two-child norm also contributed to the rapid decline in female sex ratio among children.

Population growth, especially in countries like China and India, became a matter of global concern since the early 1950s. In the 1980s an active women's reproductive rights movement coalesced around coercive population control, and the need to focus instead, on women's reproductive rights and reproductive health services. In 1994 the International Conference on Population on Development (ICPD) organised in Cairo had over 10,000 NGO participants attending, and the concept of reproductive rights and reproductive health was internationally endorsed through the ICPD Programme of Action (PoA) (Ford 2017). India was a signatory to this international agreement and promised to reform its programme.

Building an advocacy movement on population control in the State of UP and Bihar – Immediately after ICPD, the Government of India acknowledged the need for attention to informed choice in family planning and took several policy measures. The Target Free Approach to family planning was adopted in 1996. In 1999 the Government of India adopted quality of care standards for conducting family planning surgery. The National Population Policy emphasising informed choice was formulated in 2000 (Rao 2004). Uttar Pradesh (UP) and Bihar are the two most populous states in India. In 1994 when India endorsed the ICPD PoA, the total population of these two states was nearly 250 million. Despite these policy changes, observations by health activists who worked in the states of Uttar Pradesh and Bihar indicated that the situation on the ground continued to be as before. To strengthen advocacy for change at the local level, a new coalition of civil society organisations called Healthwatch UP-Bihar was formed to advocate for and monitor the family planning programme in these two states (Das 2004).

Over the next 20-year period the activists of Healthwatch UP-Bihar, later Healthwatch Forum UP and Healthwatch Bihar, continued to maintain their vigilance and undertook several activities to promote and protect the reproductive health and rights of women.

The initial task for Healthwatch UP-Bihar activists was to create a larger consensus about the deleterious impact of population control and poor-quality sterilisation services among the poor. The overwhelming opinion, created by middle class interests and the government, was that the poor were irresponsible breeders and were reluctant to adopt family planning. Several strategies were used to build a common understanding on population and health issues among civil society stakeholders. These included organising a series of consultations with different stakeholders including media persons, civil society organisations, community-based organisations, and social movements, as well as community leaders and elected representatives.

Demographic and health-related data from national surveys and those from community-based studies as well as policy and programme guidelines were simplified into fact sheets and briefs and translated into Hindi, the local language. Through a wide network of community-based observers, several adverse outcomes like repeat pregnancies after sterilisation operations, serious post-operative complications, or death during or immediately following sterilisation were identified. Fact-finding enquiries media briefings were conducted, And these activities helped build a larger coalition concerned about the issue (Healthwatch UP–Bihar 2001). Once there was enough first-hand experience about the adverse health impacts of the family planning programme, a state-level public hearing was organised in Lucknow the capital of Uttar Pradesh in 2001.

Taking the Government of India to court – No resolutions or change emerged from this public hearing. To buttress the evidence, a more systematic enquiry into the way the family planning was implemented, a more rigorous study was conducted. This study was published in EPW, one of India's leading policy journals (Das, Singh, and Rai 2004) and drew the attention of health and human rights activists. With support from human rights groups and using legal, policy, and programme standards, Healthwatch UP–Bihar led a 'public interest litigation' (PIL) in the Supreme Court of India. After two years the Supreme Court directed the states to strictly follow the quality guidelines, set up monitoring committees, and introduced the Family Planning Insurance Scheme for compensating for all adverse outcomes (Ramakant Rai vs Union of India 2003). For Healthwatch UP–Bihar this was a great assurance that things would now move in the right direction.

Things appeared to change when in 2007 the Ministry of Health and Family Welfare introduced the National Rural Health Mission. The thrust now shifted to ensuring safe maternal health outcomes. In Bihar however, the concern of population growth continued, and the family planning programme was intensified. The Supreme Court guidelines forbade temporary surgical camps, but these were popularised in Bihar. Several adverse events like infections were reported from these mass camps. Activists of Healthwatch Bihar conducted fact-finding enquiries to validate the situation on the ground. In 2012 the activists of Healthwatch Bihar filed a second PIL in the Supreme Court against such violations of health and reproductive rights. While this case was ongoing, in November 2014, 16 women died after undergoing tubal ligation in a camp in the neighbouring state of Chhattisgarh, further highlighting the continuing nature of the problem (Das and Contractor 2014). In September 2016, the Supreme Court ruled that the current practices of the family planning programme violated the Article 21 of the Indian Constitution related to the Right to Life. Once again, the advocacy efforts appeared to have given positive results (Devika Biswas vs Union of India and others 2012).

Confronting the two-child norm in Bihar – With the Supreme Court order calling for increased attention to quality of care issues, women's groups in the country started advocating with the Panchayati Raj Ministry (Ministry of Local Governments) to remove the two-child norm from those states where it existed. The Minister sent letters to all such state governments to review their laws. Since local government was an issue under state jurisdiction, the advice from the national government was not binding. Two states – Himachal Pradesh and Madhya Pradesh – amended their laws and removed the norm. It was at this point in late 2006 the activists of Healthwatch Forum Bihar noted that the Bihar government had issued an ordinance (provisional law) introducing the two-child norm into municipal elections in state. A new Chief Minister had just been elected and he promised a new era of development in the state (*The Tribune* 8 December 2006). Members of Healthwatch Bihar immediately drew the attention of several legislators to the detrimental effect of such a law before the law could be finalised. The issue was raised by opposition legislators in the State Assembly, but the law was passed without any revisions.

Having failed to stop the introduction of the two-child norm in municipal elections, Healthwatch Bihar activists focused on building a larger coalition to prevent such a norm being introduced in the gram panchayat or village-level elections. Here the scale and impact would be far more widespread. The first step was to bring activists together. As the norm affected women's participation in elected local bodies, groups working on women's leadership joined the issue immediately. This helped to bring other social movements and community groups together. A broad-based coalition called Jan Adhikar Manch (People's Rights Forum) was formed through the facilitation of Healthwatch Bihar.

The coalition used several strategies in their advocacy campaign. These included district and sub-district consultations and press conferences, sit-in demonstrations in the capital city, and a state-wide postcard campaign. The postcard campaign, like the online petitions of today, encouraged individual voters and local leaders to send postcards to their elected representatives in the state legislature asking them to stop introducing the norm. Local newspapers reported the many press conferences and other events, building a larger public opinion against the introduction of this norm. The true measure of success of this campaign between late 2006 and early 2008 is that the state of Bihar even 15 years later does not have the two-child norm in its panchayat law.

Population policies and communal demography – The Total Fertility Rate (TFR), an important metric for policy planners, has been declining steadily in India. The overall support for a population control norm has also declined. In 2014, the Bhartiya Janata Party (BJP), a Hindu majoritarian political party, came to power at the national level. Religious polarisation between Hindus and Muslims emerged as an important political strategy. In 2018, Assam, a state in the Northeast of India where the BJP was in power, introduced the two-child norm on the premise that it would help eradicate illiteracy and poverty among Muslims (NDTV 2021). The assumption being that Muslims have more children and that holds up their development. In 2021 it was proposed that the two-child norm be further extended to include eligibility for government jobs and government welfare schemes.

On 11 July 2021, the Chief Minister of Uttar Pradesh, also from BJP, announced a new population policy for the state of UP (The Hindu 2021). A two-child law was also proposed. With the state elections due in 2022, the announcement of this law was expected to deepen political polarisation along religious lines. The Healthwatch UP activists immediately started discussions on the adverse impact of such a law. This time the focus was shifted to the detrimental effects of population control laws on the welfare and rights of youth. UP had a very large number of youths who were potential voters in the upcoming election (Das 2021). It was argued that if the two-child norm was introduced and sterilisation certificates used as a means of verification, then not only would the law lead to adverse health impacts and affect the sex ratio adversely, but the birth rates could also rise as couples had their two children in quick succession. District-level consultations were held and several local newspapers, both print and digital, reported these deliberations. Posts and podcasts were also shared widely on the social media. One indirect measure of success of this advocacy was that even though the government proposing the law won the elections, no such law has been enacted till the time of writing.

Reflections from advocacy practice

This 20-year advocacy journey highlights some interesting lessons for advocacy.

Formal human rights standards and everyday practices are often at variance – in India, as in many other post-colonial countries, society is riven by many deep divisions which are very old. Despite progressive constitutions and commitments to international human rights standards these hierarchies continue to influence the way policies are implemented. Human rights relate to a redistribution of power. This redistribution is challenged by traditional customs and practices, resulting many human rights violations.

Advocacy is an iterative process; it needs ongoing review and restrategising – The case study from India clearly highlights how the logic of maintaining power and social control changes over time. To counter this dynamic policy arena, advocates need to be aware of the changing circumstance and recalibrate their strategies accordingly. And since it can be really long drawn it has to be iterative to bring about long-lasting change.

Effective advocacy requires effective communication and alliances – At its heart, advocacy is aimed at influencing public interest for change. This change is not intuitively understood or immediately supported by those in positions of power. The moral and legal dimensions are important but often not sufficient to convince many stakeholders. Effective communication strategies addressing the concerns of different stakeholders is essential to create the compulsion that strengthens arguments as well gains supporters.

Affected communities have a key role in advocacy – Women's groups were at the forefront of advocacy against population control in India and elsewhere in the world. In both UP and Bihar, the advocacy lead was taken as health rights groups and women's rights groups joined the struggle. Due to extreme poverty and strong feudal and patriarchal traditions, the women who were the most affected had the least 'voice' or ability to speak out, be heard or influence. Building a strong 'voice', especially among the most marginalised and affected communities, may require focused mobilisation for these communities to overcoming generations of internalised subordination. In a subsequent advocacy struggle by Healthwatch Forum UP for safe maternal health services, women from the community increasingly played a leading role in the advocacy struggle (Dasgupta 2011). The empowerment of the marginalised can have long-lasting impacts.

The case study from India highlights that advocacy for health rights can be a lengthy process, featuring both small and large victories as well as setbacks. The success of advocacy depends upon the openness of political regimes and policy platforms. But across the world such regimes are increasingly becoming illiberal. Health advocates need to make common cause with other activists, since rights are inter-related. The reality of human rights advocacy in the international arena is very different from what happens within countries and at the point of policy and programme implementation. Human rights advocates thus need to be continually in touch with the lived reality of communities and make them key players in the process. Human rights activists need to work closely with social activists who work with communities, and marginalised communities need to be mobilised and empowered so that they themselves can confront their own realities and decide their own destinies.

Strategies for community activism

The two cases just described and the other examples discussed elsewhere in this volume like the People's Health Movement (Chapter 2 and Chapter 5) or the Treatment Action Campaign (Chapter 2 and Chapter 6) highlight different approaches and strategies used in community activism. Community activists often draw their strategies intuitively, but many specialised schools and seminal books have helped sharpen their skills. Highlander Folk School in Tennessee was particularly influential in training activists of the civil rights movement in the US. The Coady Institute in Nova Scotia, Canada trains community leaders from all over the world. For health activists the International People's Health University (described in Chapter 5) is a useful resource. By training young health professionals and activists in the politics of health, it offers an alternative space for organising, learning, sharing, building solidarity and thinking creatively about solutions to some of the contemporary health challenges.

Some books that have been very influential include *Rules for Radicals* by Saul Alinsky and Paulo Freire's *Pedagogy of the Oppressed*. The training guide *Helping Health Workers Learn* by David Werner and Bill Bower has been a vital resource for health educators and community health workers, offering techniques and aids for participatory education and people-centred healthcare.

Published in late 2023, the book *Practical Radicals: Seven Strategies to Change the World* provides a helpful and practical synthesis on strategies for community activism. Authors Deepak Bhargava and Stefanie Luce draw upon extensive literature, their own experience in community organising as well as insights from other practitioners and present a very practical conceptual framework for developing operational strategies. Several contemporary examples, mostly from the US, including the Black Lives Matter and Occupy, are analysed.

The authors conceptualise social activism as a struggle of the 'underdog' against the 'overdog'. Strategies for any social activism need to be developed after there is a clarity about the purpose of change. There also needs to be an understanding of how power is used by 'overdogs' and how it can be deployed by the 'underdogs' to facilitate change. They recognise a tension between the need for immediate 'pragmatic' changes and a longer term 'utopian' vision for change. Strategy according to the authors are means to change the existing power relationship between the affected groups and the authorities, who have far fewer resources at their disposal. They provide an operational classification of six forms of power. These are ideological, political, economic, military, solidarity, and disruptive. This framework can be used by activists to assess their own strengths as well as that of their opposition and to develop strategies. The authors posit that activists use 'conjunctural analyses', or an understanding of social, political, economic factors, their interplay and the opportunities at any point in time, to build their strategies.

The seven strategies that the authors distil are not new propositions but another framework for consideration by social activists. The foundational act of mobilisation or constituency building is considered '*base-building*'. Activities that hurt the interests or 'wound' those in positions of power are called '*disruptive movements*'. Building a new logic for the desired changes so

Figure 8.3: The sandwich strategy – opening from above meets mobilisation from below

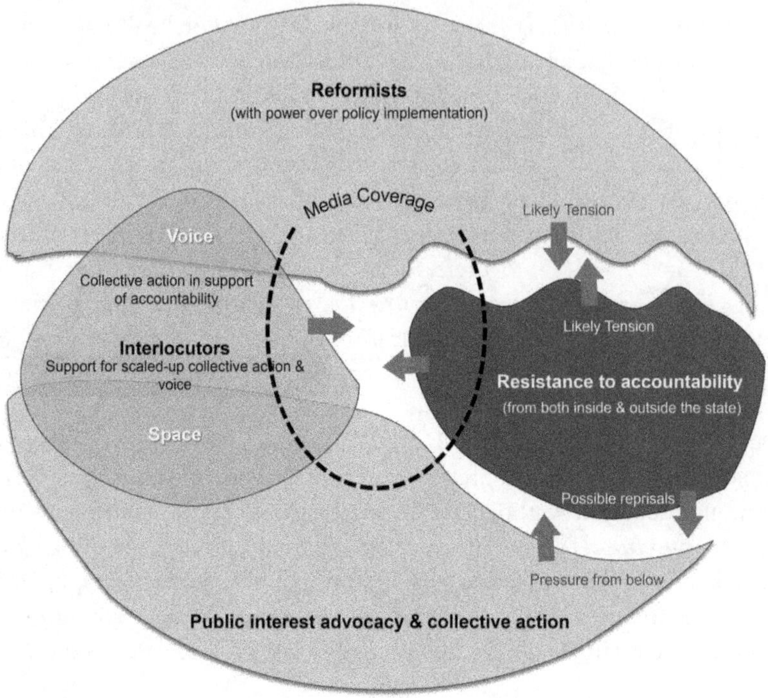

Reformists
(with power over policy implementation)

Media Coverage

Likely Tension

Voice

Collective action in support
of accountability

Likely Tension

Interlocutors
Support for scaled-up collective action &
voice

Resistance to accountability
(from both inside & outside the state)

Space

Possible reprisals

Pressure from below

Public interest advocacy & collective action

Note: Redrawn: Fox 2014. License permissions: Creative Commons (4.0)

that more people can identify is causing a '*narrative shift*'. Movements also engage in '*electoral change*' by participating in political processes. '*Inside-outside campaigns*' engage with sympathetic insiders and policy processes that are amenable to their influence along with activities in the external domain. Multiple strategies used together can build further '*momentum*'. This can lead to the change issue becoming owned by multiple stakeholders who then act out of their own convictions. The seventh strategy is not externally oriented. '*Collective care*' and collegial support between and for affected communities and community activists is crucial for the success of movements.

Jonathan Fox of the Accountability Research Centre at the American University has worked extensively with social movements in Latin America. After reviewing social accountability related activism across several countries in Asia, Africa, and Latin America he proposed a practical framework for civil society activism and advocacy which he calls the 'sandwich strategy' (see Figure 8.3). The framework recognises that while policy announcements are bold, the implementation often does not live up to the mark. According to him it is not a choice to engage in activism or advocacy, but there is a need for both. There is often a 'trigger' event like a crisis or disaster, like the COVID-19 pandemic, or a change of government or international agreement, like the ICPD. These lead to spaces or openings for bringing in some changes either in the domain of public policy or in civil society understanding and mobilisation. This provides further opportunities for civil society to engage in collective action, within formal spaces and outside them. These actions are met both by roadblocks and sympathisers who can help amplify the need for change, finally leading to some powershifts (Fox 2014; Fox and Robinson 2023).

These conceptual and operational frameworks resonate well with the examples in this chapter as well as the approaches outlined in Chapter 5.

Conclusion

This chapter provides a broad sweep of community activism in health through an exploration of several examples and broad strategies. These provide perspectives on the objectives, genesis, and conditions under which such movements can develop. While many contemporary health-related movements are dominated by a focus on diseases and drugs, there are many movements, especially in the Global South, that aspire to simultaneously improve access, systems, and wider determinants of health, and adopt strategies that go beyond lobbying and protests. We hope this chapter provides the reader with sufficient guidance to explore and engage with health focused social movements in their own practice and scholarship.

9

The role of arts, social media, and participatory action research in advancing health rights

Actor and civil rights activist Raiford Chatman 'Ossie' Davis once said that 'Any form of art is a form of power; it has impact, it can affect change – it can not only move us, it makes us move'. These famous words epitomise the power of arts and their role in organising for change. A range of different tools and tactics have been used to organise communities and advance health rights. Among these, the approaches which have shown a lot of promise are the arts, social media, and participatory action research. In this chapter we examine these tools for their potential for change, alongside the limitations and challenges in utilising these in the struggle for health justice. We illustrate both the potential and risks of these tools, offering a number of examples of promising practices from the field.

Using the arts within community development

The arts have long played a role in community development (Sjollema and Hanley 2014). This includes theatre, films, visual art/photography, music, and dance. While music and arts are increasingly utilised in popular culture to raise critical consciousness of issues (for example, climate crisis, women's rights, and so on) there has been a longer tradition of using the arts to organise, build, and sustain resistance movements and empower communities. The diverse objectives that arts can serve in bringing about social change are visualised in Figure 9.1.

The first of these is framing an issue. Framing is the meaning assigned to a specific issue and the struggle and how it is understood by participants (Adams 2002). It has aided activists in trying to attract and influence media coverage, win political support, constrain movement opponents, and influence policy makers. The Scottish Mental Health Arts Festival, which one of the authors has been engaged in, is a powerful example of this (see www.mhfestival. com). The festival has become a major national cultural event and one of the largest of its kind. Over 300 events each year including theatre, film, concerts, exhibitions, dance, comedy, literature, and fusion events have attracted audiences totalling 200,000 people. Coverage has been extensive and positive in the press, radio, and television, with an emphasis upon high-profile artists

Figure 9.1: Objectives of using the arts to achieve social change

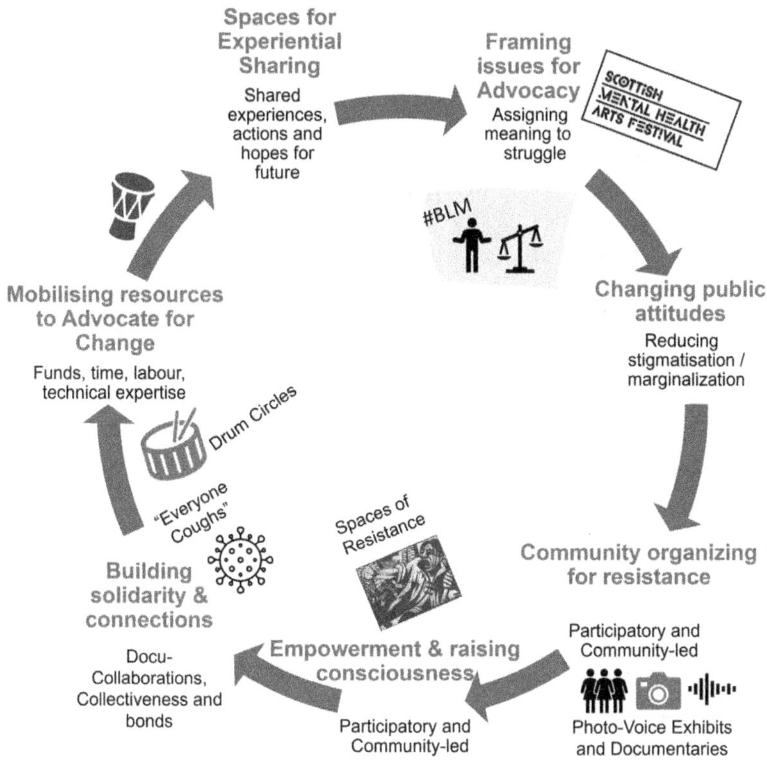

that appear at the festival. An evaluation of the festival demonstrated positive impact on the relationship between arts and mental health (Quinn et al 2011).

Arts are also an effective way to reduce stigmatisation and marginalisation of minority groups. The power of arts in raising awareness of stigmatised issues or its liberatory potential in confronting discrimination has been evidenced in the case of HIV/AIDS (Ruthven 2016) or and among young people using substance (Ritterbusch 2016). A number of studies that examined the impact of arts-based interventions on the reduction of stigma toward people with HIV found that such interventions increase public awareness and knowledge about HIV and improve attitudes of the general public and at-risk populations (Gatt, Raykov, and Vella 2021).

Community arts can be a tool for social transformation, informed by theories of empowerment and liberation (Kasat 2013). The theory and practice of community arts has been linked to activist movements for civil liberties and human rights and to liberation theorists, such as Paulo Friere and Augusto Boal (Adams and Goldbard 2002). Several studies highlight the potential for the arts to promote empowerment (or self-empowerment) among individuals and communities (Seda and Chivandikwa 2014; Massó-Guijarro, Pérez-García, and Cruz-González 2021), and facilitate liberatory experiences where communities experiencing oppression find a voice. In Wrentschur and Moser (2014), theatre was regarded as a privileged tool that could be used to empower young people, helping them to become involved in efforts to solve problems, adopting attitudes of self-confidence and self-assurance. Community arts create civic spaces for disadvantaged communities to have a voice and tell their story (Adams and Goldbard 2002). An illustration is the experience of women living with HIV in Tanzania (Harman 2016) whose testimonials formed the basis of a video documentary film called *Pili*. The project offered a voice for women and helped to gain a greater understanding of the socio-economic risks they face on a day-to-day basis (Harman 2016).

The arts can construct spaces of resistance, where individuals can engage their communities, produce collective voice, and become empowered as social actors (Vélez-Vélez and Villarrubia-Mendoza 2019).

The arts can also strengthen the agency of participants and lead to community-led advocacy and mobilise protest. The right to protest is a crucial manifestation of freedom of expression, and often takes the form of an objection to human rights abuses. Art has a long history of chronicling human rights abuses, and providing a unique form of naming and shaming, witnessing, and accountability. It is important to recognise that art and storytelling have had a much longer history in the colonised world, in revolting against oppression. For example, music and poetry have been used in anti-colonial movements in the Global South as well as in the North as a resistance tool. Street theatre has been particularly utilised for consciousness raising, organising, and resistance by activists – including within the People's Health Movement. In Scotland, the People's Health Movement used the 'theatre of the oppressed' technique with affected communities within a public hearing to enable people with lived experience of homelessness and unemployment to testify on their experiences and impact on mental health.

The arts is also used for affecting social change as it helps build solidarity and connections with other movements. These connections are essential for sustaining momentum and movements. We've seen that most powerfully in the HIV/AIDS human rights campaigns. Music, for instance, can create solidarity, as can dance and street festivals.

Art also keeps people engaged in social movements by creating a feeling of group unity and collective identity and creation of insiderness. They also help advance human rights struggles by communicating with larger society and communicating internally. Religious songs in the civil rights movement served as a communications bridge between students, the Black community, and outsiders and provided an important symbol for the struggle. We saw a similar role of the arts in Eastern Europe before the fall of communism.

Finally, the arts can support advocacy efforts through emotional engagement. Arts can stir up emotions that are useful to human rights struggles in several of the outlined ways. Song can allow people to express feelings, such as excitement and fear, and as such can be more effective than speech. We saw that powerfully in the civil rights and anti-apartheid struggle. The arts can help remove emotions such as fear or despair, which may hinder human rights actions and resistance. Perhaps most importantly, they can be a source of strength, courage, and hope for a better future. They can be critical conduits for sustaining movements by effectively reinforcing energies and creating collective effervescence, which can be important for the success of movements.

Criticisms in the use of the arts

Using art as a community development tool can also pose risks to movement building including the absence of ownership of the group process/project by community members (Carey and Sutton 2004; Purcell 2007; Ikemire 2010). The 'top-down' approach (Ikemire 2010, p 36) can position a project to be 'co-opted to serve the agenda of the people in power and thereby continue the disempowerment of the direct stakeholder group' (Purcell 2007, p 117).

The arts can also be criticised for placing too much emphasis on the individual position of the oppressed, which can lead to victim blaming. For example, migrant mothers acting out a scene in which they must convince a GP that they are entitled to see a doctor. Reducing the framing of oppression to a single antagonist may not be the most effective way to create critical conscious societies and get marginalised groups see health inequities on a structural and institutional level. If arts are to be powerful in promoting social change, they should aim to trigger social movements by empowering participants in social activism (Dalrymple 2006) and linking individual lived experiences to wider structured and systemic issues.

Emotionally charged scenes run the risk of promoting pathology and paternalism. The arts and theatre in particular can risk engendering emotions of sympathy and depiction of marginalised groups as needful as opposed to a critical and demanding of rights. Suffering of excluded communities may increase if the advances in awareness and empowerment generated by projects are not accompanied by an effective focus on the social determinants of health (Massó-Guijarro, Pérez-García, and Cruz-González 2021). For example, too much focus on material forms of development is too narrow to accommodate critical issues to modern development such as democracy, human rights, and dignity (Durden and Tomaselli 2012).

We now describe some promising examples from international practice of using different art forms, including theatre, photography, video, poetry, music, and visual art (illustrated in Figure 9.2).

Theatre is the most common art form used for community development and social change. There is a long history of using theatre as a method in community development (Ikemire 2010). 'Applied Theatre' (AT) refers to the practice of drama and theatre-based activities outside the formal school curriculum and traditional theatre buildings. It includes a range of theatre techniques and drama-based activities, projects, or interventions with a focus on providing awareness and provoking a response to social issues (Dalrymple 2006). Most of the strategies put into play in applied theatre (documentary-theatre, forum theatre, rainbow of desire, legislative theatre, street theatre) are anchored in the participatory Theatre of the Oppressed pioneered by Brazilian theatre-maker Augusto Boal (2015), Which, in turn, is inspired by Paulo Freire's Pedagogy of the Oppressed (1970). While the uses of the theatre are diverse, they all combine the political, the educational, and the social, as Freire (1970) points out with his concept of critical consciousness. Theatre has been used in a variety of settings for different purposes; for example, performance used as a transformative health rights education and empowerment strategy in a female prison in Malawi. Women prisoners devised a play using 'Theatre of the Oppressed' concepts that depicted health and prison situational injustices and trained prisoners as actors; They performed these situations,

Figure 9.2: Art in action – examples of promising practices

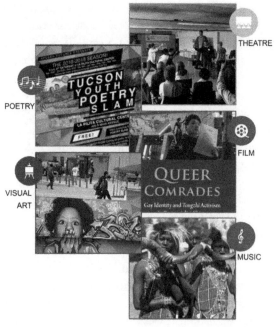

Original Image credits:
- Poetry: *Tucson Youth Poetry Slam Poster for 2018-19 used by TYPS for its Social Media Profile Covers*
- Visual Art: *Graffiti on buildings in Columbia, Bogota photographed by Eitan Abramovich for Getty Images and sourced from The Guardian.*
- Music: *Image by Washington Onyango at Nkoilale Primary School's performance at 2022 Kenya Music Festival in Kisumu for The Saturday Standard*
- Film: *Original Book Cover: Queer Comrades 2018 (Hongwei Bao) by NIAS Press*
- Theatre: *Forum Theatre at the 2nd UK People Health Assembly (Scotland)*

which the whole prison audience (facilitators, women prisoners, prison officials, policy makers) discussed and generated solutions.

Films and documentaries are another powerful medium that have been used in community development for social change (Potash 2011) and for influencing public health policy change. The power documentary films wield lies not only in the finished film itself, but in the process of collaboratively producing the film. The individuals, organisations involved in the process, and their networks help take the messages in the film off the screen and onto the streets. These larger social-issue networks, along with mass media coverage, use the documentary film to shape public opinion around an issue and are an instrumental tool in a broader social movement framework to impact change. For example, Michael Moore's 2007 documentary Sicko, portraying the dismal state of the American healthcare system was heavily covered in the press and inspired national and international demonstrations rallying for improved healthcare (Holtz 2007; Tanne 2007). Another impactful example is 'I, Daniel Blake', a 2016 film directed by Ken Loach, which is a powerful representation of the dehumanising bureaucracy of the benefits system and the impact of the cost of living crisis. It tells the story of a middle-aged man from a deprived area of the UK who is failed by the denial of health and social welfare structures. The film was used in different ways in Scotland (including screenings at the human rights festival) and the UK to highlight the effects of austerity policies and organise communities in the struggle for health rights and justice in Scotland.

Box 9.1: 'Queer Comrades' LGBTQ health activism using film

Founded in 2007, Queer Comrades is an independent LGBTQ video-streaming website that aims to document queer culture and raise LGBTQ awareness in China. It uses digital video (DV) documentaries for health communication among China's LGBTQ communities, to promote LGBTQ rights while also educating the public. Queer Comrades is not the first, or the only, LGBTQ media platform in China to use digital media to engage in health activism. It is, however, one of the most successful organisations that consciously and effectively uses DV documentaries for health education, community building, rights advocacy, and public education. The Queer Comrades webcast site excludes stigmatised, negative, and 'othered' representations of homosexuality and celebrates positive and diverse self-representations of LGBTQ people in China. By producing DV films, and by using the digital platform to engage the community and the public, Queer Comrades has gone beyond a community NGO and has started to have an impact on China's media ecology and society (Bao 2019)

Music: Given its mass appeal, music is the art form that has the potential to reach the greatest numbers of people and has often been used as a community development tool (Dillon 2007). For example, 'Krip-Hop' is a music collective developed in the US for artists of colour with disabilities. Krip-Hop is intersectional advocacy in the form of music, joining the Black community and disability community in solidarity. It challenges society's racist and ableist views, criticising police brutality, racial profiling, and the barriers that disabled Americans face on a daily basis (Gavieta 2020). Many contemporary musicians are engaging in music with social and political messages, which support community action via festivals and events. One excellent example of this is the Kenya Music Festival. The festival is an annual event featuring zonal, divisional, district, and provincial competitions leading to a national competition (Van Buren 2011). While it is explicitly an artistic development of students and of Kenya's cultural heritage, the competition also features 'special compositions' (songs and recited verses) on set themes designed to educate the audience (for example, HIV/AIDS). Leading up to the festival, student groups rehearse and perform pieces in their schools and communities.

Poetry is discussed in the community development literature as a tool for social action, most often in group settings. For example, Cohen and Mullender (1999, p 19) describe a poetry group composed of homeless individuals whose purpose was to counter the 'oppressive nature of homelessness'. A number of authors (Cohen, Johnson, and Parry 1997; Mazza 2007) also discuss poetry groups whose purpose, in part, was to raise consciousness and to collaborate for social change. Social action groups also usually participate in readings and publication as a means of reaching the larger community (Cohen, Johnson and Parry 1997; Cohen and Mullender 1999; Fisher 2003). In their analysis of an exploratory, qualitative research study carried out with 12 respondents in Montreal, Canada, who participated in community-based creative writing groups, Sjollema and Hanley (2014) found that poetry groups made a positive contribution to community building and development. The study documented the resilience of community-based poetry groups and their ability to engage marginalised populations in a process of self-expression, community building, and engagement with the wider community (Sjollema and Hanley 2014). Jocson (2006) also made the connection between youth poetry and political action in her analysis of June Jordan's Poetry for the People (P4P) programme.

Box 9.2: Youth Slam Poetry Project, Arizona, US

This project sought to understand youth voice and knowledge in their conceptions of youth rights expressed through slam poetry. It was motivated by a desire to listen and learn from youth in order to better understand their perspectives on youth, sexuality, health, and rights (YSHR). Tucson youth poetry slam (TYPS) began in 2010.

The project was interested in the creative ways youth participated in poetry slams to address this legislative climate in relation to YSHR. TYPS took place monthly as a performance poetry event in a local coffee house, culminating in a championship each year. Slam poetry was one vehicle for youth to collectively speak out about – and resist – reactionary policies on yshr, paving the way for a coalitional consciousness and collective action. With this awareness and criticalness, the youth have chosen to respond to regressive policies and practices with activism and through slam poetry. Youth voice through slam poetry exemplifies an approach that positions youth as having the knowledge to identify and speak their needs. It also highlights the critical and creative ways youth are actively engaging in the civic realm.

Visual art, in its different forms, including paintings, digital and pop artwork, and photography, is an increasingly popular method in community development (Purcell 2007) and organising for health justice. It can be an engaging group process involving community and an effective means for raising awareness of an issue with the general public. Visual art is an intervening 'facilitator of social change' in activism campaigns (Everhart 2012). This view approaches art from a representational perspective, a tool to be wielded by social actors with the particular intention of producing an image of self. For instance, art assists in the construction of 'self-representation and the production of meaningful identities', which support a sense of collectivity and solidarity (Mahon 2000). Visual art allows people to present themselves [to others] visually providing the tools for the articulation of their own representations (Cushing and Drescher 2009).

Box 9.3: Photography to counter stigma surrounding street-based substance abuse in Colombia

A long-term participatory action research (PAR) initiative started in 2008 with a group of street-connected female and transgender adolescents. The PAR initiative developed a project focusing on inhalant/glue and bazuco addiction (the 'Beyond Glue and Bazuco' project). The research design of the 'Beyond Glue and Bazuco' subproject included semi-structured life history interviews and cartographic focus groups with street-connected adolescents who have consumed glue and/or bazuco since early childhood. Following the research, participants designed participatory photography and video to counter stigma and discrimination, which was used to advocate for change with policy makers, involving a presentation of the participatory video, a presentation of life histories led by street-connected adolescents and a collective viewing of participants' photographs in a gallery posted on the wall of the auditorium. After the forum, an NGO was established, which campaigned for youth sex workers' health rights, developed a human rights project with street-connected and LGBTQ populations in prison, and a participatory photography project with street-connected youth involved in prostitution.

Arts-based, creative methods have found resonance and success in engaging with marginalised communities. One innovative method is photovoice. Photovoice is 'a process by which people can identify, represent, and enhance their community through a specific photographic technique' in which participants take pictures that are meaningful to them (Wang 2003). During the subsequent interviews, participants reflect on the meaning of the images and critically discuss the strengths and weaknesses of their social or physical environment represented in the photographs. Finally, they advocate for change by communicating what the pictures revealed to those who influence programme development and policy (Wang and Burris 1997). Photovoice has been used to empower people in countries including India, China, the UK, and the United States (Jurkowski and Ward 2007; Kapilashrami and Marsden 2018) by enabling disadvantaged groups to critically reflect on their photographic images, express their social experiences, and use the consciousness toward taking action (Wang and Burris 1997).

The role of mass media and social media

Mass media refers to media technologies used to disseminate information to a wide audience. Its key function is to communicate various messages through television, movies, advertising, radio, the internet, magazines, and newspapers. Social media are defined as forms of electronic communication through which users create online communities to share information, ideas, personal messages, and other content (such as videos).

Mass media and social media serve various functions in the public health arena. They are an important source of health information and provide novel opportunities for citizens to access information on diagnosis and treatment that enables them to manage their health. They can be used for education and awareness raising about a specific health issue for which they have higher risk factors – for example, on how to practice safe sex for LGBTQ+ individuals or raise awareness of mental health issues among young people (Halsall et al 2019).

It can also be effective in promoting health literacy and healthy practices and can draw attention to inequities in access to healthcare for marginalised groups, supporting campaigns for more accessible health services. Social media can also bring communities together to seek mutual support on health and provide a platform to exchange ideas on different health issues affecting any population or group (Moorhead 2013). Those who self-identify as having specific health conditions can build communities, curate and share narratives of illness, treatment, and recovery, and raise their profile in order to attract funds and lobby for research. An example of this is from Ghana, where the news media's advocacy on tramadol and codeine abuse helped build a campaign advocating for policy actions by the government to address the social and public health impact of tramadol and codeine on communities (Thompson and Ofori-Parku 2021). These forums have also been utilised to organise, strengthen, and sustain collective action.

Two promising examples from the practice of grassroots movements that serve as powerful conduits of raising critical consciousness, building collective solidarity towards social change, are the Khabar Lahariya Dalit women's-run newsletter in India and the use of citizens' media in Brazil (see Box 9.4 and Box 9.5).

Box 9.4: Khabar Lahariya journalist collective, India

Khabar Lahariya, or 'Waves of News', is an all-women journalist collective led by Dalit women in India. Khabar Lahariya has trained local women from underprivileged communities as journalists and reported on hyperlocal issues often overlooked in the mainstream press. The organisation's work – spanning parts of two of the country's poorest states, Uttar Pradesh and Madhya Pradesh – has exposed environmental degradation caused by illegal stone mining, ensured delivery of public services like healthcare in isolated villages, showcased the vibrancy of rural life, and helped rape victims get justice by questioning police inaction. Over the years, the group has trained about 500 rural women in journalism. Its current team of 20 reporters includes women who were never formally educated, were survivors of domestic violence, and a former child worker at the local stone quarries. A documentary on their crusading journalism, 'Writing with Fire', was shortlisted for the Oscars in 2022 (Masih 2022).

Box 9.5: Citizens' media in the favelas, Brazil

Citizens' journalism has been used in community development to improve access to health services for low-income communities. Viva Favela, a digital journalism project, was initiated in the favelas (unincorporated neighbourhoods that have grown up alongside Brazil's major metropolitan areas) of Rio de Janeiro. The project developed digital news content generated by favela residents for its website.

The first strategy of Viva Favela was built around training classes in digital photography and blogging to produce material for a central website, www.vivafavela.com.br.

Designed to house news reports, personal essays (mini editorials), and photographs by favela residents trained by staff members, the site provided a modest attempt to promote 'empowerment through self-representation'. The project expanded its base of users, and the site became fully interactive. After registering, users gained the ability to upload photographs with text through a customised phase of Flickr and to upload video through an embedded YouTube interface. The initiative captured the personal narratives of people living in the favelas, which helped to raise consciousness of the public health concerns facing these communities and debunk stereotypes around favelas. It also led to collective action in supporting a campaign for improved health service provision and tackling the underlying social and environmental issues that resulted in poor health outcomes within the favelas (Davis 2015).

Critiques of mass and social media in community development and health practice

There are several criticisms of using the mass media and social media as a campaign tool for community development. First is the focus on the individual rather than structural dimensions of inequalities in health. Creating a campaign around people's personal narratives of health conditions runs the risk of individualising the problem, in that it puts the responsibility on the shoulders of the individual to navigate the inequities they face, rather than seeing the causes of the health issue as socially and politically determined, described as the social determinants of health (Marmot and Wilkinson 2005). Mass media campaigns, especially utilised for public health, are often framed within the Western notion of personal choice and responsibility. This limits its effectiveness in guaranteeing structural reforms necessary for social change (Berg, Harting, and Stronks 2021). Second, while the media can be used to create empathy and understanding, this does not guarantee advocacy and activism, let alone the desired social change. There is the question of whether social media allows the longevity necessary for social movement building, which requires developing a collective and shared vision as well as shared politics. This can be seen in awareness raising using social media, which often leads to what has been termed 'slacktivism'. This refers to a desire to perform a token display of support for a social cause accompanied by a lack of willingness to invest significant effort for meaningful change (Glenn 2015). As such, arguments against social media's effectiveness propose that without organisation and face-to-face interaction, social media are not enough to sustain a protest movement (Smith, Krishna, and Al-Sinan 2019). In addition, the growth of digital media has undermined the power of many health campaigns. Digitalisation has meant that the bottom-up, grassroots efforts of early health activism has been replaced in many cases with a more top-down version with activists taking less of a role than in the past in constructing meaning. Petersen and colleagues (2019) argue that digital media and bio-digital citizenship has fundamentally reoriented 'activism'; wherein online platforms are used more to raise profile of issues and create support groups of communities experiencing similar conditions than to advance struggles for rights.

Most notably, the digital divide and inequities in access to technologies have implications for who has access to information. Thus, the true potential of social media and technology can only be reached with improving access and capacities to utilise these.

While different forms of media have been used in health advocacy, we focus on the role of social media.

Using social media as a health advocacy tool to influence decision-makers and build coalitions for change

Social movements utilise social media as a community development tool to organise campaigns, disseminate information, share lived experiences, and advocate for change. Engaging in advocacy and affecting real political pressure and subsequent policy change require several different elements within community development practice. Social media is often deployed to frame an issue, generate a sense of urgency, and build credibility of a specific campaign. Social media can offer spaces for individuals to 'resist and challenge dominant political or cultural discourse and foment the idea of a "right time" for change' (Rodriguez 2013). Social media gives minority groups an avenue through which they can rebuke, alter, or control the dominant media narrative. There are many examples of local marginalised groups taking advantage of social media to shape discourse about health disparities. For example, migrant construction workers in Singapore produced TikTok videos sharing their structural, social, and health conditions during the pandemic (Kaur-Gill 2022). Through the production of short videos, workers detailed the precarities they faced during the pandemic, making visible their dormitory conditions, stringent medical surveillance of their bodies, mobility restrictions imposed on them, and the mental health impacted by confinement and isolation. They also customised the platform's editability features to produce and edit vernacular content for entertainment and information-sharing, and digitally archived their precarities on the platform. By generating this content, workers responded to the exclusions they faced in the host country, undoing the mainstream discursive silencing of their lived experiences as subaltern workers in the city-state. Workers' use of TikTok presents opportunities for activism and organising that effect change.

Social media communities play a crucial role in 'collectivising' around a single issue and facilitating direct participation in specific campaigns. For example, social media campaigns from the civil rights movement and the #BlackLivesMatter movement inspire other marginalised communities learning how to utilise social media to facilitate community action and frame events. A particular strength of social media is its reach. It helps to build transnational and translocal connections, thus not only broadening the movements' base but also the scale at which these issues can be tackled. Social media enables the direct participation of communities in social movements through live streams, real-time tweets and postings, hashtag campaigns, and virtual petitions. These methods enable communities to feel involved in and engage with wider campaigns: the immediacy of social media means they can observe, react, and interact with people from all geographic areas. Using social media communities affected groups can create supportive communities, recognise common struggles and help a movement's audience grow both in terms of number of participants and increased understanding through wider exposure. A strong example of this is the #bombadeinsulinaalAUGE movement in Chile (see Box 9.6).

Box 9.6: #bombadeinsulinaalAUGE movement, Chile for improved access to insulin

In Chile, patients with Type 1 diabetes led the #bombadeinsulinaalAUGE. Specifically, people with type 1 diabetes and their families organised themselves around demand for improving access to insulin. The campaign pressurised the government of Michelle Bachelet (2014–2018) to incorporate an insulin pump into the universal health cover plan that provided healthcare for this chronic condition. They organised an 'online march' that sought to position #bombadeinsulinaalAUGE as a trending topic, building a social network with support of influencers, followed by an online petition addressed to the then Minister of Health and raising public support for the same. The campaign strengthened its use of social media, showing the support of different TV actors, journalists, and athletes. #bombadeinsulinaalAUGE was able to achieve its goal, ensuring that a national-level health policy incorporated universal coverage (González-Agüero et al 2022).

Another powerful aspect of digital and social media's role in health advocacy is its ability to organise communities as well as different stakeholders and constituencies. There are many examples of social media use to foster collaboration with stakeholders such as non-government organisations (NGOs), advocacy coalitions, social media influencers, and respected/ popular public and political figures to raise the profile and appeal of causes. These stakeholders are strategically deployed to pressurise governments to engage in policy dialogue change (Ramirez et al 2021; González-Agüero et al 2022). A powerful example of mobilising communities is the

Caremongering movement that emerged to address health and social needs during COVID-19 (see Box 9.7).

Box 9.7: Caremongering movement in Canada

Following the outbreak of the COVID-19 pandemic in March 2020, Canadian communities began a Facebook social media movement, #Caremongering, to support vulnerable individuals in their communities. Local #Caremongering Facebook groups formed to help provide vulnerable individuals in their communities with access to food, services, information, and other necessities. Member volunteers deliver supplies and food, donate goods, run errands, or do chores for those quarantining. A study of the #Caremongering Facebook groups found that the volunteer social media initiative spread to at least 130 communities, engaging over 190,000 Canadians within days of the COVID-19 emergency declaration (Seow et al 2021). These groups spread to every province and territory across Canada. Convening for a shared purpose over social media is a powerful means by which communities can address complex problems that cannot be resolved without shared responsibility of individual citizens and joint action. Such organising, fuelled by social media, can be an important public health tool to support the health of vulnerable populations in the community.

Finally, it has been argued that social media not only enables communication and organisation within a movement, but also helps diversifying the repertoire of strategies (Theocharis et al 2015) employed in social change efforts. For example, social media has played an important role in the 16 Days of Activism against Gender-based Violence, resulting in a wide array of strategies being used by the movement, including simultaneous actions and flash mobs across the world. Effective campaigns utilise multiple media platforms such as social media and local/national news, increasing the publicity about and reach of the issue (Jain et al 2021), forging political alliances, and forcing real political change (Eke et al 2021).

Participatory research

Participatory research emerged in recognition of the importance of power relations in the research process and thinking differently about the construction and use of knowledge. It represents a set of values and principles in which the community determines the research agenda and jointly shares in the planning, implementation of data collection, and analysis and dissemination of the research (Wallerstein et al 2003). It served as an alternative way to interpret and describe social reality from the perspective of the 'knower' or 'knowledge holder'. Some delineations of participatory research (for example, participatory action research) go beyond interpretation and have the intent of transforming that reality 'with' and 'by' not 'for' the oppressed.

Participatory research views knowledge as socially constructed and raises the question of who defines knowledge, about whom and for what purpose. Informed by the emancipatory traditions of critical and feminist theories, researchers adopt more reflexive and pluralistic modes of inquiry. Habermas proposes using critical or emancipatory reason, which reflects the research aim to go beyond existing power struggles, such as ethnic and religious strife and understand why a situation has occurred and how it can be addressed, which fits well with a Global South Freirean perspective (Wallerstein et al 2003). Friere (1970) argues that emancipatory knowledge can lead to having the power to make change.

The historical development of participatory research

There are many reasons why participatory research approaches gained greater prominence. Tandon (1996) highlights a number of historical influences on the development of participatory research approaches.

One such influence was debates within the sociology of knowledge, which presented alternative views of human history from the point of view of the marginalised, poor, and weak as opposed to the dominant form of knowledge produced and articulated from the point of view of the powerful (Doyle McCarthy 1996). A second important influence was the practice of adult education in countries of the South, which led to a reformulation of research that was influenced by the principles of adult education. The work of Ivan Illich and Paulo Freire was very influential. Illich's critique of schooling in modern societies and Freire's contribution to alternative pedagogy became the basis for linking participatory research as an educational process with the framework of popular education. In the Global South, especially Latin America, Asia, and Africa, *participatory research* was driven by the structural crisis of underdevelopment, the radical critiques of existing theory, liberation theology, and the search for a new, engaged practice in the adult education and development fields in how best to work with communities vulnerable to the impact of globalisation (Stern 2019). There was a transformation in how knowledge creation was understood, which was driven by Latin American academics. Rather than knowledge emanating from the academy, value was placed on knowledge based on lived experience. Paulo Freire (1970), through his book *Pedagogy of the Oppressed*, influenced the transformation of the research relationship from viewing communities as objects of study to viewing communities as subjects of their own experience and enquiry. Rather than viewing research as neutral, practitioners of participatory research were committed to critical consciousness, emancipation, and social justice. The core premise of such engagement was that communities would transform their environment through their own praxis.

A third major influence on participatory research methodologies was the work of feminist theorists. Historically, feminism and feminist researchers have challenged the hegemonic male-centric (that is, Western, White male) patriarchal gaze on social reality prevalent in research paradigms. In doing so, feminist scholars offered a strong critique of the limits of the knowledge and methods created from the perspective of elite white men's experiences referring to it as 'partial and even perverse understandings of social life' (Harding 1987, p 7). While acknowledging the potential of participatory research, feminists argued that as an alternative paradigm PAR was not free of the male biases inherent in mainstream research design and practices, often rendering the issues and experiences of women and gender power relations invisible. In essence, feminist theory and praxis remained peripheral to early developments in participatory research (Hall 1981; Tandon 1988) and have over the years enriched this field in several ways. These include (1) aligning research methodologies with a feminist theoretical perspective that bring gender power relations and empowerment into sharp focus, (2) bringing centre-stage the political nature of research, and (3) requiring the researcher to be acutely aware of the inequities, exclusions, and abuse of power that characterise societies and human interactions (including researcher-community) (Maguire 1987). Such feminist perspectives can both reveal entrenched inequities in societies, while creating opportunities for greater balance of power and emancipatory knowledge seeking (Harding 1986; Collins 1990; Reid 2004). Since feminisms include diverse schools of thought – liberal Marxist, radical, postmodern, Black, postcolonial, intersectional among others – the field of PAR benefitted from developments within these fields, in the process enhancing its emancipatory and decolonising potential (Darroch and Giles 2014). For instance, PAR has been integrated with intersectionality and utilised by feminist researchers to examine health inequalities in accessing community assets and to action a collective agenda for tackling the social determinants of mental health (Kapilashrami and Marsden 2018, see Scottish PHM case study in Chapters 3 and 5).

Core concepts of participatory research approaches

Participatory research places critical consciousness, emancipation, and personal and societal transformation as the core defining principles of research. A key underpinning concept is participation, discussed in Part I of this book. In the health field, international conferences including Alma-Ata (1977), Ottowa (1986), and Jakarta (1996) have highlighted the importance of community participation to improve health conditions. Participation is seen as crucial because it enables communities and health professionals to understand each other's concerns, ensures cultural sensitivity of programmes, and responsiveness to local community needs, and protects health rights. Despite participation being valued, questions remain on the authenticity of the process and whether the reality/practice of participation reflects the rhetoric and ideals.

An understanding of power relations is central to participatory approaches (see Figure 9.3). Although knowledge is a major source of power and control, other power relations are also central for understanding the dynamic relationships between researchers/facilitators and communities. These include the societal context in which research takes place, the origins of the research and the purpose of the research itself. Participatory researchers who want to address inequalities, need to produce knowledge that clarifies and seeks to change the unequal distribution of power and resources within society. Foucault (1982) argued power is productive and relational,

Figure 9.3: Rights-based participatory approach

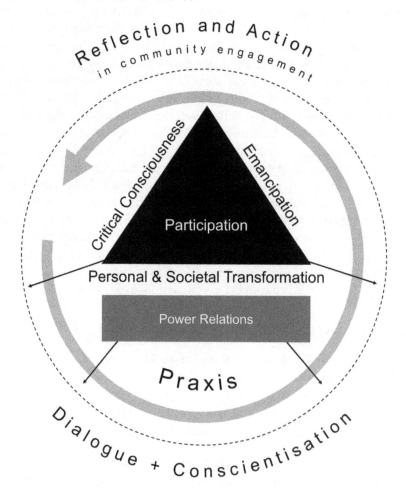

conceptualising power as being built into a web of discourses and practices found in institutions, communities, and practices that are exercised through actions in a multiplicity of relationships. Participatory research challenges communities to reshape their self-view away from clients or consumers toward democratic community participation and participatory research.

The final defining aspect of participatory research is the emphasis of praxis, that is, learning from the practical application and actions in the community. This concept is inspired by the work of Paulo Freire's concern for the powerless through his efforts to teach literacy in the favelas and barrios with the marginalised poor in Brazil. Freire generated dialogue to facilitate transformation to conscientisation (or critical consciousness) and praxis (action based on critical reflection). To Freire, the purpose of education is human liberation, which means people are the subjects of their own learning, not empty vessels filled by the knowledge of experts. The goal of dialogue and conscientisation is praxis, the interaction between reflection and actions people take to promote individual and social change. The Freirean popular education approach is creative in that it presents findings in ways participants can see their reality on a physical form (using pictures, videos, role plays and so on). Different communication methods such as photovoice and Theatre of the Oppressed are expressions of this approach. Popular education has been applied in the fields of adult education and community development globally.

Participatory research in practice

Case study 9.1: Challenging austerity and examining intersectional inequalities in access to health resources in disadvantaged communities: the cases of Scotland and Eastern Europe

A promising example of participatory research is from the tradition of feminist PAR. Researchers adopted an innovative approach combining intersectionality and PAR that was operationalised in three overlapping phases with disadvantaged communities in Scotland. The objective was to examine the distribution and access to health resources, as defined by communities in two deprived neighbourhoods. A preparatory phase helped establish relationships with participant groups and policy stakeholders, and challenge core assumptions underlying the study design. Field-work and analysis was conducted iteratively in two phases: with a range of participants working in policy and community roles (or 'bridge' populations), followed by residents of two Edinburgh localities with relatively high levels of deprivation. Traditional qualitative methods (interviews, focus groups) alongside participatory methods (health resource mapping, spider-grams, photovoice) were employed to facilitate action-oriented knowledge production among multiply disadvantaged groups. This was achieved by employing visual and arts-based methods to map local assets in the community (see

Figure 9.4), by the communities, and sharing lived experiences of barriers to accessing these. As the study progressed, communities experiencing multiple structural exclusions and disadvantages were involved in a collective and democratic space of knowledge building that culminated in a public hearing on the social determinants of mental health and well-being. The hearing included forum theatre performed by the affected communities to testify on the violations of their health rights, and the social determination of their mental health. The process also enabled movement building for health rights, engaging communities and groups in the Scottish People's Health Movement. The participatory process also led to the development of people's health manifestos that were utilised as tools to lobby political parties and advocate for a healthier Scotland. For instance, Kapilashrami (one of the authors) was involved in delivering sessions on health inequalities at annual conferences of political parties (such as the Green Party) that informed their party manifestos and engaging other parties through policy dialogue and hosting events.

Members of the COPASAH network in Eastern Europe have used participatory research with Roma people in countries like Bulgaria and Macedonia. COPASAH is a global community of practitioners using participatory approaches to social action in the field of health. The Roma are among the most marginalised communities in Europe. Many of the organisation working with Roma are Roma-led and have built their own capacities through partnerships with each other and other COPASAH members. Over the last ten years, members used various tools such as community mapping, interviews with health providers, exit interviews with health users, testimonies, photovoice, community score cards and others to highlight health problems faced by the community. Some of the achievements include greater awareness of health-related entitlements among Roma communities and improved interactions with service providers. This resulted in improvements in immunisation rates of Roma children, better maternal health services, and improved health insurance coverage, among others.

These are just a few examples of the use of participatory research, which continues to be a growing field of practice.

The potential of participatory approaches may however be limited by several factors that can be grouped under technical or practical, conceptual, and accountability challenges.

Since participatory research processes hinge on mutual trust, shared purpose, and action, they are necessarily slow and require long-term commitment, funding and perseverance on all sides. Since the process is iterative it can also falter and may need to be re-built. Costs of building trusting relationships and re-building supporting processes and structures are not built-in, short-term research and development projects.

Further, assessing the impact of participatory processes using mainstream evaluation or (research) impact assessment tools can be counterproductive

Figure 9.4: Participatory resource map of Leith, Edinburgh prepared by young, 2nd generation girls from minoritised ethnicities participating in a PAR study

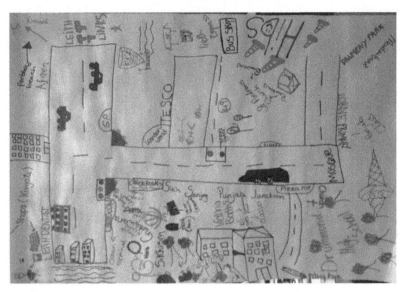

Source: Kapilashrami et al (2016)

and antithetical to the core ideas of participation as 'process'. Top-down approaches in both research and development practice often tend to incorporate participation as an after-thought or add-on to other methods, as a means to validate findings or increase community's acceptability of the policy/programme introduced. Evaluating success of participation requires a more robust understanding of incremental changes and the ability to see the benefit of small changes brought about by participation, at individual, household, community or institutional level, and over time. There is also the inconsistency or varying degree to which core progressive tenets of participatory approaches are incorporated in research and practice. This may relate to the fuzziness and the different meanings the concept and process of participation generates. For instance, even though it depends on shared purpose, the practical gains and motivations of the researcher/facilitator and the community may differ. While the researcher/facilitator may be interested in the fidelity of processes, the community members may require effective services. Equally, the inconsistency in adopting transformative aspects of participatory research may arguably result from the absence of a coherent theoretical framework. While participatory research is influenced by critical and feminist theory, not all participatory research confronts unequal power relations or achieves dismantling of hierarchies in society. In fact, Wallerstein (1999) has argued that such equilibrium of power can never be achieved in CBPR. Postcolonial scholars on the other hand have argued that both the dominant Western discourse and practice of CBPR are embedded in a colonial and imperialist paradigm that 'embodies the potential for an unjustified exercise of power' (Cooke and Kothari 2001, p 4). Research and researchers can thus serve to reproduce these hierarchies unless being conscious of, transparent about, and accountable to confronting these power dynamics.

Conclusion

This chapter has demonstrated the tremendous value of the arts, social media, and participatory research as community development tools for advancing health rights. In terms of future directions for research, the challenge going forward is how to effectively gather evidence on the impact of these initiatives as well as learning from the process of engaging and empowering communities. There is an increasing need for community development practitioners to explore how arts, social media, and participatory research can be used to advocate for change, and the enabling conditions under which these result in change. These approaches should ultimately be judged on their ability to contribute to community capacity building and changes in health inequalities. In the pursuit of community health and development as well as social justice, communities must be empowered to catalyse, deliver, and ultimately sustain change and these are important tools in helping to achieve this.

10

Conclusion: Community organising and collective action as countervailing power for healthy and just societies

What do the COVID-19 pandemic, the humanitarian crisis, and a fast-depleting planet or the climate crisis all have in common? That these are some of the major threats or crises facing the world today? Or that these are reflective of social injustices on a grand scale. And that any response to these must bring to the fore a systematic understanding of the neglect, the actions and inactions that have contributed to these crises, and the power relations that determine where the impact is most felt. The unprecedented human suffering (experiences of illness, deaths, and divided societies) resulting from these injustices disproportionately affect the disadvantaged and socially marginalised populations.

Who are these people? As described in the book, they are the rising precariat class disenfranchised because of rising inflation, cost-of-living, depleting health, and other public services, as well as rapid technological changes that they do not have the resources to use or adapt to. They are the 'othered' and oppressed due to their subordinate caste or religious minority status. They are the 120 million people forcibly displaced and rendered homeless due to wars, conflicts, and persecution, and the 10 million that are rendered stateless, denied a nationality and accompanying basic human rights. They are the people living in the 'deep end'[1] – in favelas, in detention camps, in islands that are at risk of sinking or coastlines exposed to cyclones and tsunamis. They are the Black and other ethnic and religious minorities who die prematurely from police brutality or in crossing borders, the indigenous who are deprived of their own land and resources, the migrant women whose bodies are used as guinea pigs for contraceptive experiments and to meet family planning targets.

They are at once the drivers of economic growth – essential for sustaining economies amid recession and inflation, working in farms, plantations, construction, service sector as frontline workers, and the objects of racial scapegoating, hate, and violence. The riots and extremist attacks on asylum seekers and religious and ethnic minorities that engulfed the UK and other European cities are a manifestation of this hate. They are the feared 'other', the 'outsiders' who threaten all that the insiders or the privileged hold dear – their land, their jobs, their public resources, their security, their health. They are also the 'carriers of disease' in times of pandemics, abandoned and forcibly confined to spaces of containment, surveillance, and incarceration.

Why are we here?

The central premise advanced in this book is that the neoliberal state and market forces – and the colonial legacies that underpin these – have unleashed unrivalled economic growth and wealth creation. This has resulted in unprecedented human suffering and an emotional psycho-social crisis, and an unparalleled atomisation of contemporary societies.

Our society has become increasingly atomised, characterised by individualism and what Pankaj Mishra in the *Age of Anger* refers to as a 'brutish struggle for existence and recognition (that) has come to define individual and geopolitical relations across the world' (Mishra 2017, p 328). Individuals in these modern societies are subsumed in ideas of self-protection, self-preservation and self-empowerment and are moving away from public life and civic spaces. The constant influx of fake news fueled by far-right narratives has also resulted in chronic mistrust, othering, and an overall lack of empathy to the growing suffering of others. Such atomisation limits any progress towards full realisation of health rights and the desired goal of just societies.

The promise of technology and healthcare innovations is stymied by the asymmetry of markets and the growing socio-economic divide with the rich getting richer and the poor getting poorer. Such inequality is associated with a whole range of poor health and development outcomes that have made SDGs and public health goals a distant reality for people. Against this backdrop, the gap between what people want and what governments are delivering has led to widespread anger and frustration. Equally pervasive is the anger and despair arising from the indifference of political leaders who have turned their back on people and are complicit in spreading the discourse of scapegoating and fear mongering. The resulting loss of political, social, and economic power and personhood while palpable, is also what drives people to act. People are no longer mute spectators of oppressions. Through mass uprisings and sustained protests they are calling attention to diverse dimensions of the poly-crises, and for rebuilding societies and a just world. It is in these actions and resistances, and the praxis it generates, that we locate the central theses of this book.

Countering this loss of political and economic power demands a strong countervailing power from below

To change the prevailing regressive trends, we argue, it may be necessary to create countervailing power. The idea of countervailing power relates to the dispersion and expansion of political power across society, that is, power to the people. John Kenneth Galbraith introduced countervailing power in the context of corporate governance and economic power to refer to power that is both 'public, in the form of a strong regulatory state, and private, in the form of labor unions and consumer cooperatives' (Galbraith 1954). In the context of health governance, private power takes the form of organised collectives at the grassroots and demands a strong *independent* regulatory state. Such power may provide the leverage needed to question authority without fear of reprisal, and to get those in power to take cognisance of people's lived realities, protect their rights as well as the political space necessary for grassroots resistance to the depredations of neoliberal capitalism. Such alternative experiments of state-power can be seen in the examples described in book, where community organising and actions strengthened state welfare role, and led to more effective people-centred, rights-based solutions.

However, the development of countervailing power needs a certain minimum opportunity and capacity for organising. Further, 'power to the people' in an atomised world of deep inequalities and ideological divisions may not level the playing field. Nor would the gains be equally distributed in the community. As discussed in Chapter 4, participation that fails to attend to positions of marginality and precarity risks privileging the already powerful and thereby widening inequalities and divisions. Thus, building countervailing power in the contemporary world requires a different politics of activism and organising. We propose three concrete ideas here:

First, empowering individuals to exercise their agency and voice is insufficient. *Empowerment of the collective is necessary to achieve collectively defined goals and vision.*

Such an approach to empowerment demands radical ideas for how we organise communities, in all its diversity. The idea of a collective must go beyond the societal divisions and identity politics that are a product of colonial, neo-colonial, and neoliberal rule. These divisions lead to conflicting struggles and claims or 'Oppression Olympics' that pits marginalised communities against each other for claims over finite resources and opportunities.

To counter the divisiveness that characterises our society, *we urgently need alternatives to current mainstream organising approaches.* As discussed in Chapter 3, much organising and action is driven by people that come together around shared interests, issues, or concerns linked to a defined place/geography or identity. The alternatives *demand building alliances across single issue struggles and utilising specific causes and struggles as entry points to strengthen wider movements tackling the syndemics of poly-crisis.*

Organising in this sense is not only a *means* to countervail power. *Rather, empowered and critically conscious collectives that arise from such organising may themselves be the countervailing movement necessary to dismantle and reverse power.* In other words, collectives that are empowered, aware, connected, and share a vision for constructive social change can derive the social and political power that is necessary for exercising agency at multiple levels. Members of the collective may exercise individual agency in the choices they make in their daily lives around health or their role as conscious citizens in the community. They may be stronger advocates for reforms needed at institutional level to realise these health choices (for example, Green General practices in the UK, better work conditions of nurses and junior doctors), and bring wider change in consciousness at societal level (against unjust wars, patients over profits). We saw this multi-level change in the land reforms movements in Brazil, as well as the organising around the gas leak in Bhopal. In the latter, communities simultaneously tackled harmful commercial practices, sought state, market, and investor accountability, and linked the disaster with wider environmental concerns, while seeking compensation for the health of affected persons and monitoring industries. The broad-base health activism of the PHM that has triggered bottom-up health advocacy through health manifestos and public hearings while linking with local struggles is also a case in point.

Second, the *countervailing power and action must be firmly located in intersectional justice and global solidarity*. This is essential to effectively subvert the current global crises including health injustice. We discussed in Chapter 5 the threat of atomisation and siloed actions as core challenges to building and sustaining health movements today. Such atomisation as described deepens the tensions between the politics of recognition and representation and the politics of distribution. To counter this we need *radical shifts in our approach to resistance and our actions of solidarity*. Actions that can unite across our differences, build bridges across seemingly disparate struggles, and build a social order that is conducive to promoting, precipitating, and sustaining the necessary change.

We need solidarity among different groups, including communities in the North and the South, between diverse struggles and campaigns, and those experiencing multiple injustices. For example, patients organising around health rights and violations, health professions demanding improved conditions of work and pay, and activists addressing backlash and threats to civil liberties must stand together. We also need solidarity between those suffering acute injustices and those who are empathetic but not directly oppressed. Most crucially, we must deepen affective links between these groups to combat the divisive discourses and foster constructive social change. While campaigns may continue to target specific threat – health, the environment or other determinants – movement building requires influencing values and relationships. The success of social movements, as argued in Chapters 5 and 8, depends on building collective care and solidarity among affected communities and health activists. Above all, there is a pressing need to *build communities of Trust, communities of Hope and communities of Solidarity*.

Intersectional justice approach can be a powerful tool for organising and activism based on principles of solidarity. Applied to health this lens helps us recognise the interconnections between the economic, socio-cultural, and political spheres of distribution, recognition, and representation that drive health inequalities and health injustices experienced in societies. This iteration of intersectionality is not about individual identity positions and politics, but the wider gendered, colonial, neoliberal systems that create these marginal identities. The purpose of this tool goes beyond identifying who is most vulnerable to ill-health – but recognising and organising around the interconnected systems of oppressions that create these vulnerabilities.

Awareness raising, a critical part of organising and empowerment initiatives, in this context cannot be limited to increasing knowledge of entitlements among the most affected and disenfranchised. Community development and health activism needs targeting everyone on the social gradient and raising consciousness about power, privilege and oppression. It also merits drawing attention to the syndemic conditions that underlie the different injustices linked to the poly-crisis defined at the outset.

Finally, *health justice is a useful entry point for organising and collective action for social justice.* Actions to achieve good health and well-being takes us to the fundamental conditions and resources for health. The *Ottawa Charter for Health Promotion* (WHO 1986) identified these as: peace, shelter, education, food, income, a stable ecosystem, sustainable resources, social justice, and equity. Addressing these conditions and securing these prerequisites for all can lead to healthy individuals and societies. In other words, improving population health and challenging health inequities – the objectives of health activism – can be a useful and less contested entry point for affecting the interconnected systems that are driving poly-crisis and therefore wider social change. For example, campaigns targeting vaccine apartheid and universal access to medicines have prompted reforms in trade and economic systems and facilitated reforms for effective governance and greater international cooperation. The book has offered insights into a range of advocacy strategies and tactics utilised to demand reforms in healthcare, frame health as rights and not a commodity or a good, and realise the indivisible rights to social, economic, political, and environmental determinants of health. From organising symbolic protests and demonstrations, to concerted lobbying and advocacy to influence institutions and policies are some of the tactics to resist forces that threaten health and social well-being. These are powerful actions that have long-lasting impacts on our environment.

As we look back at COVID-19, we find innumerable examples of extending solidarity and support to affected people, irrespective of their class and other societal divisions. Food kitchens run by minority faith institutions for all, transporting oxygen cylinders across to those in need, offering food and shelter to migrants, to name a few. The pandemic also made visible the plight and social inequalities experienced by specific population groups who were otherwise invisible or peripheral to social welfare planning. The case of internal migrants and refugees we discuss in Chapter 8 is a notable example. As their struggles – loss of livelihoods, wages and in some cases lives – came to light, this triggered targeting social security and relief measures to these populations. Organising on health issues and engaging health communities can therefore be a powerful medium for building bridges between activism of asserting marginal identities and activism for apolitical common goods. The book offers useful insights into the longstanding history of health based social movements that have organised communities for action, advocacy, and activism. These have served as powerful conduits of social change, but change brought about by dismantling power structures that have created the conditions for people to die.

The book provides several examples and a variety of strategies for organising and addressing health issues. The ideas and practices illustrated in this book serve two purposes. First, we hope that they inspire action and facilitate the transfer of the ideas and tools discussed in the book for organising for social change in other parts of the world. Since people worldwide are experiencing common problems, threats, and resisting in distinct ways, learning from successes and challenges, and adapting strategies across socio-economic and country-level contexts can strengthen the practice of rights and justice. Second, while describing our experiences, we attempt to generate praxis-based theoretical positions and ideas (not a grand meta theory) for those interested in how change can happen and how health rights can be realised. We reflect on our own experiences and learnings of movements, community organising, and action – in both Global North and South – and situate these in scholarship and theories, creating a generative space for dialogue. This is a humble attempt to correct the epistemic injustice evident in the disconnect between sites of knowledge and sites of action/practice that has characterised global health justice and participatory development scholarship to date. We hope that these ideas are a modest contribution to our joint effort towards a healthier and more just world.

Glossary

Aid effectiveness agenda

a generic term used to refer to both the discourse and practice of improving the degree of success of international aid in meeting development goals, and a broad consensus on what is needed to produce such success. Improving transparency and accountability of donors and recipients are key cornerstones of the agenda. A series of global initiatives was launched between 2005 and 2015 – in milestone conferences in Paris (2005), Accra (2008), Busan (2011) – calling for more effective cooperation and coordination of international aid. The Addis Ababa Action Agenda (2015) endorsed at the international conference on financing for development and the Global Compact (2017) also endorse key principles of aid effectiveness, laying a foundation to support the implementation of the 2030 Sustainable Development Agenda.

Critiques of the aid effectiveness agenda in development abound, encompass the top-down and euro-centric orientation to setting targets; weak internalization of its founding principles by donors and recipients and reluctance to change practices on the ground (Brown 2020); overwhelming thrust on accountability to donors, less towards citizens (Kapilashrami 2010); as well as the politics of aid that are unaccounted for in aid effectiveness debates.

Anti-science movement

a group of people who reject scientific methods and ideas, and instead believe in pseudoscience and conspiracy theories.

Complexity theory

a framework that helps to understand and transform healthcare systems by acknowledging that they are complex and constantly changing.

Conscientisation

a process of developing and strengthening consciousness, especially critical awareness of social reality.

Decolonisation   refers to the process of gaining political and economic independence from foreign rule through an active transfer of power. Such power transfer occurs not only through military and administrative withdrawal of foreign powers and establishing sovereign rule, but by rebuilding institutions and knowledge systems that are free from the cultural and social effects of colonial era violence, racism, and Eurocentrism and of economic colonial practices of wealth extraction.

Decoloniality   a perspective or praxis that involves an ongoing 'undoing' of colonisation and its legacies to create more just societies.

De-growth   a critique of capitalist growth that emphasises organising the economy around human needs rather than capital interests.

Empowerment   is understood as the process by which those who have been denied the ability to make strategic life choices gain that ability.

Epistemic   relating to knowledge or the study of knowledge.

G-20 countries   an intergovernmental forum that includes 19 countries, the European Union (EU), and the African Union (AU).

Habitus   the way that people perceive and respond to the social world they inhabit.

Hegemony   the dominance of one group or perspective. the social, cultural, ideological, or economic influence exerted by a dominant group.

International Covenant   international legal instruments which, in international law, legally bind those States that choose to accept the obligations contained in them.

Intersectionality   the interconnectedness of social categories, such as race, gender, class, sexuality, and ability, and structural conditions – all of which shape an individual's experiences and opportunities.

Millennium Development Goals
the United Nations Millennium Development Goals (MDGs) are eight goals that UN Member States had agreed to try to achieve by the year 2015. The United Nations Millennium Declaration, signed in September 2000, committed world leaders to combat poverty, hunger, disease, illiteracy, environmental degradation, and discrimination against women. The MDGs were derived from this Declaration. Each MDG had targets set for 2015 and indicators to monitor progress from 1990 levels.

Neo-colonial
a type of imperialism that involves a state indirectly controlling another state that is nominally independent.

Neo-liberal
a political and economic philosophy that emphasises free trade, deregulation, globalization, and a reduction in government spending.

Ontological
the philosophical study of being.

Pedagogy
the method and practice of teaching, especially as an academic subject or theoretical concept.

Poly-crisis
a situation in which several crises occur simultaneously or in close succession and influence or reinforce each other.

Post-colonialism
the historical period or state of affairs representing the aftermath of Western colonialism.

Post-growth
an economic philosophy that recognises the limits to growth on a planet with finite resources.

Post-structuralism
an intellectual movement from France during the 1960s and 1970s that challenged the belief in stable or unchanging meanings and identities.

Praxis
the process of free, creative, and critical reflection upon action to transform the world and its defining contexts. Stems from the ideas of Greek philosophy that knowledge and actions are interconnected and should be combined to achieve meaningful change.

Precarity
a state of persistent insecurity induced by failing social and economic networks of support.

Primary Health Care
primary health care is essential health care based on practical, scientifically sound, and socially acceptable methods and technology made universally accessible to individuals and families in the community through their full participation and at a cost that the community and country can afford to maintain at every stage of their development in the spirit of self-reliance and self-determination. It forms an integral part of the country's health system, of which it is the central function and main focus, and of the overall social and economic development of the community. It is the first level of contact of individuals, the family, and community with the national health system bringing health care as close as possible to where people live and work and constitutes the first elements of a continuing health care process.

Sustainable Development Goals
the Sustainable Development Goals (SDGs), also known as the Global Goals, were adopted by the United Nations in 2015 as a universal call to action to end poverty, protect the planet, and ensure that by 2030 all people enjoy peace and prosperity. The 17 SDGs are integrated – they recognise that action in one area will affect outcomes in others, and that development must balance social, economic, and environmental sustainability. Countries have committed to prioritise progress for those who are furthest behind. The SDGs are designed to end poverty, hunger, AIDS, and discrimination against women and girls.

Syndemicity

the idea that diseases occur within specific environments (physical, social, biological and psychological) and result from a constellation of factors. Also used to refer to the interaction between diseases and their underlying conditions that influences vulnerability and severity.

Universal Health Coverage

universal health coverage means that all people have access to the health services they need, when and where they need them, without financial hardship. It includes the full range of essential health services, from health promotion to prevention, treatment, rehabilitation, and palliative care.

Notes

Chapter 1

[1]   We see the influential work of the knowledge commissions on social determinants, and on political and commercial determinants as critical for the paradigm shift in these understandings.

Chapter 3

[1]   Settlement activities were part of a reformist settlement movement that began in the 1880s and peaked around the 1920s in the UK and the US. The object was intermixing of classes by establishing 'settlement houses' in poor urban areas, in which volunteer middle-class workers would live in proximity to their low-income neighbors. The intent was that sharing of knowledge and culture, and provisions of services such as daycare, language classes, and healthcare would improve the lives of the poor in these areas.

Chapter 5

[1]   This is based on a talk delivered by Kapilashrami at the 2014 'Health in Action' conference organised by Medact. For more details, see:
        https://www.medact.org/2014/resources/videos/health-in-action-recordings/
[2]   For details on the process through which PHM informs these global health governances initiatives, see: Narayan (2006), Baum and Fisher (2010), Baum et al (2020), Ashraf et al (2023).
[3]   For more detailed review of donor-led public private partnerships and commercialisation of healthcare in LMICs, see Hamer and Kapilashrami (2020).

Chapter 10

[1]   Deep end metaphor is used to refer to the socio-economically most deprived areas and was inspired by Tudor Hart's seminal piece in 1971 that highlighted the presence of inverse care law in healthcare. The inverse care law suggests that the availability of good medical care has an inverse relationship with the need for it in the population served.

References

Abbasi, K. (1999) Free the slaves. *BMJ*, 318: 1568–9. https://www.ncbi. nlm.nih.gov/pmc/articles/PMC1115949/pdf/1568.pdf

Abraham, M.-R. (2020) Gandhi and green democracy: The evolution of eco swaraj. https://vikalpsangam.org/article/gandhi-and-green-democracy-the-evolution-of-eco-swaraj/

ACLED (2021) A year of COVID 19: The pandemic's impact on global conflict and demonstration trends. https://acleddata.com/acleddatanew/wp-content/uploads/2021/04/ACLED_A-Year-of-COVID19_April2021.pdf

Adams, J. (2002) Art in social movements: Shantytown women's protest in Pinochet's Chile. *Sociological Forum*, 17(1): 21–56.

Adams, D. and Goldbard, A. (eds) (2002) *Community, Culture and Globalization*. New York: Rockefeller Foundation.

Aggarwal, R. and Goodell, J. W. (2009) Markets and institutions in financial intermediation: National characteristics as determinants. *Journal of Banking & Finance*, 33(10): 1770–80.

Akintunde, T. S., Oladipo, A. D., and Oyaromade, R. (2019) Socioeconomic determinants of health status in Nigeria (1980–2014). *African Review of Economics and Finance*, 11(2): 365–88.

Ali, M. (2012) Mystery of Glasgow's health problems, *The Guardian*, 6 November. https://www.theguardian.com/society/2012/nov/06/mystery-glasgow-health-problems

Alinsky, S. (1972) *Rules for Radicals: A Practical Primer for Realistic Radicals*. New York: Vintage Press.

Aljazeera (2022) Antivaccine protesters rally in France, Germany, Austria, Italy, *Aljazeera*, 9 January. https://www.aljazeera.com/news/2022/1/9/more-than-100000-rally-in-france-against-covid-vaccine-rules

Allsop, J., Jones, K., and Baggott, R. (2004) Health consumer groups in the UK: a new social movement? *Sociology of Health & Illness*, 26(6): 737–56.

Alma Ata (1977) Declaration. https://cdn.who.int/media/docs/default-source/documents/almaata-declaration-en.pdf?sfvrsn=7b3c2167_2

Ambrose, S. (2005) Social movements and the politics of debt cancellation. *Chicago Journal of International Law*, 6(1), Article 16. https://chicagounbound.uchicago.edu/cjil/vol6/iss1/16

Amin, S. (1993) Social movements at the periphery. In P. Wignaraja (ed) *New Social Movements in the South: Empowering the People*. New Delhi: Vistaar Publications.

Amnesty International (2020) Nigeria: Authorities must uphold human rights in fight to curb COVID-19, Amnesty International. https://www.amnesty.org/en/latest/news/2020/04/nigeria-covid-19/

Amnesty International (2024) Global: Dow shareholders must help ensure justice for victims of Bhopal disaster, *Amnesty International.* https://www. amnesty.org/en/latest/news/2024/04/global-dow-shareholders-must-help-ensure-justice-for-victims-of-bhopal-disaster/

Anandhi, S. and Kapadia, K. (eds) (2017) *Dalit Women: Vanguard of an Alternative Politics in India.* London: Routledge.

Anil, P. (1994) Obsession with targets. *Health Millions,* 2(3): 37–8.

Arnstein, S. R. (1969) A ladder of citizen participation. *Journal of the American Institute of Planners,* 35(4): 216–24.

Arthur, M., Saha, R., and Kapilashrami, A. (2023) Community participation and stakeholder engagement in determining health service coverage: A systematic review and framework synthesis to assess effectiveness. *Journal of global health,* 13: 04034. https://doi.org/10.7189/jogh.13.04034

Asch, A. (2002) Disability equality and prenatal testing: Contradictory or compatible. *Florida State University Law Review,* 30: 315.

Ashraf, A., Muhammad, A., Fazal, Z., Zeeshan, N., and Shafiq, Y. (2023) The role of civil society organizations in fostering equitable vaccine delivery through COVAX. *Eastern Mediterranean Health Journal,* 29(4): 232–5.

Asnarulkhadi, A. (1996) People's Participation in Community Development and Community Work Activities: A Case Study in a Planned Village Settlement in Malaysia, PhD thesis, University of Nottingham.

Assai, M., Siddiqi, S., and Watts, S. (2006) Tackling social determinants of health through community based initiatives. *British Medical Journal,* 333: 854–6.

Assies, W. (2003) David versus Goliath in Cochabamba: Water rights, neoliberalism, and the revival of social protest in Columbia. *Latin American Perspectives,* 30(3): 14–36.

Atampugre, N. (1998) Colonial and contemporary approaches to community development: a comparative overview of similarities and differences in West African experiences. *Community Development Journal,* 33(4): 353–64.

Aveling, E. and Jovchelovitch, S. (2014) Partnerships as knowledge encounters: A psychosocial theory of partnerships for health and community development, *Journal of Health Psychology,* 19(1): 34–45.

Azémar, C., Desbordes, R., Melindi-Ghidi, P., and Nicolaï, J. P. (2022) Winners and losers of the COVID-19 pandemic: An excess profits tax proposal. *Journal of Public Economic Theory,* 24(5): 1016–38.

Baines Johnson, E. L. and Bilici, İ. (2018) Participation And Development A Critical Assessment: Is Participation Vital For Development? *The Journal of International Social Research,* 11(56): 111–16.

Bajaj, S. S., Maki, L., and Stanford, F. C. (2022) Vaccine apartheid: global cooperation and equity. *Lancet,* 399(10334): 1452–53.

Balcazar, H., Rosenthal, L., De Heer, H., Aguirre, M., Flores, L., Vasquez, E., Duarte, M., and Schulz, L. (2009) Use of community-based participatory research to disseminate baseline results from a cardiovascular disease randomized community trial for Mexican Americans living in a U.S.-Mexico border community. *Education for Health (Abingdon)*, 22(3): 279.

Bao, H. (2019) Queer comrades: Digital video documentary and LGBTQ health activism in China. In V. Lo, C. Berry, and G. Liping (eds) *Film and the Chinese Medical Humanities*. London: Routledge, 188–204.

Baru, R., Acharya, A., Acharya, S., Kumar, A. S., and Nagaraj, K. (2010) Inequities in access to health services in India: Caste, class and region. *Economic and Political Weekly*, 45(38): 49–58.

Baum, F. and Fisher, M. (2010) Health equity and sustainability: extending the work of the Commission on the Social Determinants of Health. *Critical Public Health*, 20(3): 311–22.

Baum, F., MacDougall, C., and Smith, D. (2006) Participatory action research. *Journal of Epidemiology and Community Health*, 60: 854–7. https://doi.org/10.1136/jech.2004.028662

Baum, F., Freeman, T., Sanders, D., Labonté, R., Lawless, A., and Javanparast, S. (2016) Comprehensive primary health care under neo-liberalism in Australia. *Social Science & Medicine*, 168: 43–52.

Baum, F., Sanders, D., and Narayan, R. (2020) The global People's Health Movement. What is the People's Health Movement. *Saúde Debate, Rio De Janeiro*, 44(1): 37–50.

Bauman, Z. (2001) Consuming life. *Journal of Consumer Culture*, 1(1): 9–29. https://doi.org/10.1177/146954050100100102

Bayer, R. (1994) AIDS: Human rights and responsibilities. *Hospital Practice*, 29(2): 155–64.

BBC News (2020) Uganda – Where security forces may be more deadly than coronavirus. *BBC News*. https://www.bbc.com/news/world-africa-53450850

BBC (2021) COVID: Huge protests across Europe over new restrictions. *BBC News*. https://www.bbc.com/news/world-europe-59363256

Beard, R. L. (2004) Advocating voice: Organisational, historical and social milieux of the Alzheimer's disease movement. *Sociology of Health and Illness*, 26(6): 797–819. https://doi.org/10.1111/j.0141-9889.2004.00419.x

Beatty, C. and Fothergill, S. (2013) The local and regional impact of the UK's welfare reforms. *Cambridge Journal of Regions, Economy and Society*, 7(1): 63–79.

Benford, R. D. and Snow, D. A. (2000) Framing processes and social movements: An overview and assessment. *Annual Review of Sociology*, 26(1): 611–39.

Berg, J., Harting, J., and Stronks, K. (2021) Individualisation in public health: Reflections from life narratives in a disadvantaged neighbourhood. *Critical Public Health*, 31(1): 101–12. https://doi.org/10.1080/09581 596.2019.1680803

Bernstein, M. (2005) Identity politics. *Annual Review of Sociology*, 31: 47–74.

Besson, E. S. K. (2022) How to identify epistemic injustice in global health research funding practices: A decolonial guide. *BMJ Global Health*, 7(4): e008950.

Betancourt, J. R. (2007) Racial and ethnic disparities in health care. In L. Epstein (ed) *Culturally Appropriate Health Care by Culturally Competent Health Professionals*. Tel Hashomer, Israel: The Israel National Institute for Health Policy and Health Services Research, 18–32.

Bhakuni, H. and Abimbola, S. (2021) Epistemic injustice in academic global health. *The Lancet Global Health*, 9(10): e1465–70.

Bhatnagar, G. V. (2020) Delhi violence exposed holes in healthcare system, political representation. *The Wire*. https://thewire.in/communalism/ delhi-riots-health-care-system-holes

Bhattacharya, J. (2014) The genesis of hospital medicine in India: The Calcutta Medical College and the emergence of a new medical epistemiology. *The Indian Economic and Social History Review*, 51(2): 231–64. https://doi.org/ 10.1177/0019464614525726

Biswas, S. (2020) Coronavirus: India's pandemic lockdown turns into a human tragedy. *BBC News*. https://www.bbc.com/news/world-asia-india-52086274

Bloom, G., Standing, H., and Lloyd, R. (2008) Markets, information asymmetry and health care: Towards new social contracts. *Social Science & Medicine*, 66(10): 2076–87.

Boal, A. (2015) *Teatro del Oprimido*. Buenos Aires: Interzona Editores.

Bodini, C., Sanders, D., and Sengupta, A. (2018) *The Contribution of Civil Society Engagement to the Achievement of Health for All*. Cape Town: People's Health Movement. https://phmovement.org/wp-content/uploads/2018/ 07/CSE4HFA_FinalReport_Long_180909.pdf

Bonevski, B., Randell, M., Paul, C., Chapman, K., Twyman, L., Bryant, J., Brozek, I., and Hughes, C. (2014) Reaching the hard-to-reach: a systematic review of strategies for improving health and medical research with socially disadvantaged groups. *BMC Medical Research Methodology*, 14: 42.

Boydell, V., Neema, S., Wright, K., and Hardee, K. (2018) Closing the gap between people and programs: Lessons from implementation of social accountability for family planning and reproductive health in Uganda. *African Journal of Reproductive Health*, 22(1): 73–84.

Boydell, V., Schaaf, M., George, A., Brinkerhoff, D. W., Van Belle, S., and Khosla, R. (2019) Building a transformative agenda for accountability in SRHR: Lessons learned from SRHR and accountability literatures. *Sexual and Reproductive Health Matters*, 27(2): 64–75.

Brinkerhoff, D. (2003) *Accountability and Health Systems: Overview, Framework, and Strategies*. Bethesda, MD: The Partners for Health Reformplus Project, Abt Associates Inc.

Brinkerhoff, D. W. (2004) Accountability and health systems: Toward conceptual clarity and policy relevance. *Health Policy and Planning*, 19(6): 371–9.

Brohman, J. (1996) Popular development: Rethinking the theory and practice of development. Cambridge, MA: Oxford University Press.

Broughton, E. (2005) The Bhopal disaster and its aftermath: A review. *Environmental Health*, 4(6). https://doi.org/10.1186/1476-069X-4-6

Brown, P., Zavestoski, S., McCormick, S., Mayer, B., Morello-Frosch, R., and Gasior Altman, R. (2004) Embodied health movements: New approaches to social movements in health. *Sociology of Health & Illness*, 26(1): 50–80.

Bryson, L. and Mowbray, M. (1981) 'Community': The spray-on solution. *Australian Journal of Social Issues*, 16: 255–67. https://doi.org/10.1002/j.1839-4655.1981.tb00713.x

Burhansstipanov, L., Dixon, M., and Roubideaux, Y. (2001) Cancer: A growing problem among American Indians and Alaska Natives. In M. Dixon, and Y. Roubideaux (eds) *Promises to keep: public health policy for American Indians and Alaska natives in the 21st century*. Washington, D.C.: American Public Health Association.

Burke, J. (2019) Bhopal's tragedy has not stopped: The urban disaster still claiming lives 35 years on. *The Guardian*. https://www.theguardian.com/cities/2019/dec/08/bhopals-tragedy-has-not-stopped-the-urban-disaster-still-claiming-lives-35-years-on

Calvi, R. and Mantovanelli, F. G. (2018) Long term effects of access to health care: Medical missions in colonial India. *Journal of Developmental Economics*, 135: 285–303. https://doi.org/10.1016/j.jdeveco.2018.07.009

Campbell, C. (2020) Social capital, social movements and global public health: Fighting for health-enabling contexts in marginalised settings. *Social Science and Medicine*, 257: 112153.

Campbell, C., Cornish, F., Gibbs, A., and Scott, K. (2010) Heeding the push from below: How do social movements persuade the rich to listen to the poor? *Journal of Health Psychology*, 15(7): 962–71.

Campfens, H. (ed) (1997) *Community development around the world: Practice, theory, research, training*. Toronto: University of Toronto Press.

Carey, P. and Sutton, S. (2004) Community development through participatory arts: lessons learned from a community arts and regeneration project in South Liverpool. *Community Development Journal*, 39(2): 123–34.

Carroll, A. and Kapilashrami, A. (2020) Barriers to uptake of reproductive information and contraceptives in rural Tanzania: An intersectionality informed qualitative enquiry. *BMJ Open*, 10(10): e036600.

Carty, V. (2014) Arab Spring in Tunisia and Egypt: The impact of new media on contemporary social movements and challenges for social movement theory. *International Journal of Contemporary Sociology*, 51(1): 51–80.

Castells, M. (2012) Networks of outrage and hope – social movements in the Internet age. *International Journal of Public Opinion Research*, 25: 398–402.

Chancel, L., Piketty, T., Saez, E., and Zucman, G. (2022) *World Inequality Report*. Paris: World Inequality Lab.

Chandhoke, N. (2007) Engaging with civil society: The democratic perspective, Non-governmental Public Action Program, Centre for Civil Society, London School of Economics and Political Science.

Chaturvedi, S., Randive, B., Diwan, V., and De Costa, A. (2014) Quality of Obstetric Referral Services in India's JSY Cash Transfer Programme for Institutional Births: A Study from Madhya Pradesh Province. *PLoS ONE*, 9(5): e96773. https://doi.org/10.1371/journal.pone.0096773

Chattopadhyay, M. (2018) Rabindranath Tagore's model of rural reconstruction: A review. *International Journal of Research and Analytical Reviews*, 5(4): 142–6.

Chávez, V., Duran, B., Baker, Q., Avila, M. M., and Wallerstein, N. (2008) The dance of race and privilege in CBPR. In M. Minkler and N. Wallerstein (eds) *Community Based Participatory Research for Health: Process to Outcomes*, 2nd edition. San Francisco, CA: Jossey-Bass, 91–105.

Chiripanhura, B. M. and Niño-Zarazúa, M. (2016) The impacts of the food, fuel and financial crises on poor and vulnerable households in Nigeria: A retrospective approach to research inquiry. *Development Policy Review*, 34(6): 763–88.

CIVICUS (2021) Freedom of Peaceful Assembly – CIVICUS – Tracking conditions for citizen action. CIVICUS. https://monitor.civicus.org/COVID19September2021/

Cleary, S. M., Molyneux, S., and Gilson, L. (2013) Resources, attitudes and culture: An understanding of the factors that influence the functioning of accountability mechanisms in primary health care settings. *BMC Health Services Research*, 13(320). https://doi.org/10.1186/1472-6963-13-320

CO_2 Coaltion (2021) 97% Consensus: What consensus. CO_2 Coalition, 28 October. https://co2coalition.org/media/97-consensus-what-consensus-2/

Cochran, P. A., Marshall, C. A., Garcia-Downing, C., Kendall, E., Cook, D., McCubbin, L. et al (2008) Indigenous ways of knowing: Implications for participatory research and community. *American Journal of Public Health*, 98: 22–7.

Cohen, J. L. (1985) Strategy or identity: New theoretical paradigms and contemporary social movements. *Social research*, 52(4): 663–716.

Cohen, M. A., Kupcu, M. F., and Khanna, P. (2009) The New Colonialists. https://foreignpolicy.com/2009/10/07/the-new-colonialists/

Cohen, R. and Rai, S. M. (2000) *Global Social Movements*. London and Brunswick NJ: The Athlone Press.

Cohen M. B., Johnson J. M., and Parry J. K. (1997) Self-directed community group for homeless people: Poetry in motion. In J. K. Parry (ed) *Prevention to Wellness through Group Work*. London: Hawarth Press, 131–42.

Cohen, M. B. and Mullender, A. (1999) The personal in the political: Exploring the group work continuum from individual to social change goals. *Social Work with Groups*, 22(1): 8–21.

Collin, J., Hill, S. E., Kandlik Eltanani, M., Plotnikova, E., Ralston, R., and Smith, K. E. (2017) Can public health reconcile profits and pandemics? An analysis of attitudes to commercial sector engagement in health policy and research. *PloS ONE*, 12(9): e0182612.

Collins, C. (1999) 'Break the chains of debt!' International jubilee 2000 campaign demands deeper debt relief. *Review of African Political Economy*, 26(81): 419–22. https://www.jstor.org/stable/pdf/4006470.pdf

Collins, P. H. (1990) Black feminist thought in the matrix of domination. *Black Feminist Thought: Knowledge, Consciousness, and the Politics of Empowerment*, 138: 221–38.

Competitive Enterprise Institute and others (2017) Letter to President Donald J Trump. https://cei.org/sites/default/files/20170508%20 CEI%20Paris%20Treaty%20with%20logos%20-%2044%20Final.pdf

Connelly, M. (2006) Population control in India: Prologue to the emergency period. *Population and Development Review*, 32(4): 629–67.

Contractor, S. and Das, A. (2015) Does one-size-fit-all? Re-evaluating the approach to address Maternal Health of Tribal Communities in India. Paper presented at *The ghosts of MDG: Unpacking the logics of development*, the 13th Development Dialogue, ISS The Hague, November 4–5.

Cooke, B. (2003) A new continuity with colonial administration: Participation in development management. *Third World Quarterly*, 24(1): 47–61. https://doi.org/10.1080/713701371

Cooke, B. and Kothari, U. (eds) (2001) *Participation: The New Tyranny*. New York: Zed Books.

Cornwall, A. (2000) Beneficiary, Consumer, Citizen: Perspectives on Participation for Poverty Reduction, Study No. 2. Stockholm: Swedish International Development Agency (SIDA).

Cornwall, A. (2006) Historical perspectives on participation in development. *Commonwealth & Comparative Politics*, 44(1): 62–83.

Cornwall, A. (2008) Unpacking 'participation': Models, meanings and practices. *Community Development Journal*, 43(3): 269–83.

Cornwall, A. and Shankland, A. (2008) Engaging citizens: Lessons from building Brazil's national health system. *Social Science & Medicine*, 66(10): 2173–84.

Countdown to 2030 (n.d.) *A decade of tracking progress for maternal, newborn and child survival: The 2015 Report.* https://www.countdown2030.org/2015/2015-final-report

Cowan, H. (2021) Taking the national(ism) out of the national health service: Re-locating agency to amongst ourselves. *Critical Public Health*, 31(2): 134–43. https://doi.org/10.1080/09581596.2020.1836328

Cox, M. (2018) *Understanding the global rise of populism.* Strategic Update (February 2018). London: LSE IDEAS, London School of Economics and Political Science.

Crenshaw, K. (1989) Demarginalizing the Intersection of Race and Sex: A Black Feminist Critique of Antidiscrimination Doctrine, Feminist Theory and Antiracist Politics. *The University of Chicago Legal Forum*, 140: 139–167.

Crenshaw, K. (2013) Demarginalizing the intersection of race and sex: A black feminist critique of antidiscrimination doctrine, feminist theory and antiracist politics. In K. Maschke (ed) *Feminist Legal Theories*. New York: Routledge, 23–51.

Crenshaw, K. (2017) *On Intersectionality: Essential Writings.* New York: New Press.

Crossley, N. (2022) Social Movements and Health. In J. Gabe and L. Monaghan (eds) *Key Concepts in Medical Sociology*, 362.

CSDH (2008) Closing the gap in a generation: Health Inequity through action on the social determinants of health. Final report of the commission on social determinants of Health. Geneva: World Health Organization.

Cueto, M. (2018) The history of international health: Medicine, politics and two socio-medical perspectives 1851–2000. In C. McInnes, L. Lee, and J. Youde (eds) *The Oxford Handbook of Global Health Politics*. New York: Oxford University Press.

Cushing, L. and Drescher, T. W. (2009) *Agitate! Educate! Organize! American Labor Posters.* Ithaca, NY: Cornell University Press.

Cyril, S., Smith, B. J., Possamai-Inesedy, A., and Renzaho, A. M. N. (2015) Exploring the role of community engagement in improving the health of disadvantaged populations: a systematic review. *Global Health Action*, 8(1). https://doi.org/10.3402/gha.v8.29842

Dalrymple, L. (2006) Has it made a difference? Understanding and measuring the impact of applied theatre with young people in the South African context, Research in Drama Education. *The Journal of Applied Theatre and Performance*, 11(2): 201–18. https://doi.org/10.1080/13569780600671070

D'Ambruoso, L., Izati, Y., Martha, E., Kiger, A., and Coates, A. (2013) Maternal mortality and severe morbidity in rural Indonesia Part 2: Implementation of a community audit. *Social Medicine*, 7(2): 68–79.

Darroch, F. and Giles, A. (2014) Decolonizing health research: Community-based participatory research and postcolonial feminist theory. *The Canadian Journal of Action Research*, 15(3): 22–36.

Das, A. (2004) Ensuring quality of care in sterilisation services. *Indian Journal of Medical Ethics*, 1(3).

Das, A. (2017) The challenge of evaluating equity in health: Experiences from India's maternal health program. *New Directions for Evaluation*, 154: 91–100.

Das, A. (2021) Why UP's proposed population control bill is bad as policy and politics. 20 July. *Indian Express*. https://indianexpress.com/article/opinion/columns/uttar-pradesh-proposed-population-control-bill-policy-and-politics-7412610/

Das, A., Singh, D., and Rai, R. (2004) Medical negligence and rights violations. *EPW*, 39(39). https://www.epw.in/journal/2004/35/comment ary/medical-negligence-and-rights-violation.html

Das, A. and Contractor, S. (2014) India's latest sterilisation camp massacre. *British Medical Journal*, 349: g7282. https://doi.org/10.1136/bmj. g7282

Dasgupta, J. (2011) Ten years of negotiating rights around maternal health in Uttar Pradesh, India. *BMC International Health and Human Rights*, 11(Suppl 3): S4. https://doi.org/10.1186/1472-698X-11-S3-S4

Davies, J. S. (2011) *Challenging Governance Theory: From Networks to Hegemony*. Bristol: Policy Press.

Davis, S. (2015) Citizens' media in the favelas: Finding a place for community-based digital media production in social change processes. *Communication Theory*, 25(2): 230–43. https://doi.org/10.1111/comt.12069

Dawes, D. E. (2020) *The Political Determinants of Health*. New York: Johns Hopkins University Press.

De Mesquita, J. B., Lougarre, C., Montel, L., and Sekalala, S. (2023) Lodestar in the Time of Coronavirus? Interpreting International Obligations to Realise the Right to Health During the COVID-19 Pandemic. *Human Rights Law Review*, 23(1): 1–25.

Desilver, D. (2018) For most U.S. workers, real wages have barely budged in decades. Pew Research Center. https://www.pewresearch.org/fact-tank/2018/08/07/for-most-us-workers-real-wages-have-barely-budged-for-decades/

Devika Biswas vs Union of India and Others (2012) Petition No 95. https://www.escr-net.org/caselaw/2017/devika-biswas-v-union-india-others-petition-no-95-2012

Dhanraj, D. (1991) *Something Like a War* [Film].

Dillon, S. (2007) Assessing the positive influence of music activities in community development programs. *Music Education Research*, 8(2): 267–80.

Dominelli, L. (2006) *Women and Community Action* (Revised Second Edition). Bristol: Policy Press.

Dorfman, L., Cheyne, A., Friedman, L. C., Wadud, A., and Gottlieb, M. (2012) Soda and tobacco industry corporate social responsibility campaigns: How do they compare? *PLoS Medicine*, 9(6): e1001241.

Durden, E. and Tomaselli, K. (2012) Theory meets theatre practice: Making a difference to public health programmes in southern Africa. Professor Lynn Dalrymple: South African Scholar, activist, educator. *Curriculum Inquiry*, 42(1): 80–102.

Duvendack, M. and Sonne, L. (2021) Responding to the multifaceted COVID-19 crisis: The case of Mumbai, India. *Progress in Development Studies*, 21(4): 361–79. https://doi.org/10.1177/14649934211030449

DW (2022) Thousands protest Covid curbs across Europe, 9 January. https://www.dw.com/en/thousands-protest-covid-curbs-in-europe-amid-omicron-surge/a-60374676

Edelstein, D. (2010) The Super-Enlightenment: Daring to know too much. *Studies on Voltaire and the Eighteenth Century*. Oxford: Voltaire Foundation.

Edgman-Levitan, S. and Cleary, R. D. (1996) What information do consumers want and need? *Health Affairs*, 15(4): 42–56.

Edwards, G. (2004) Habermas and social movements: what's 'new'? *The Sociological Review*, 52(1_suppl): 113–30.

Egan, M., Abba, K., Barnes, A., Collins, M., McGowan, V., Ponsford, R., Scott, C., Halliday, E., Whitehead, M., and Popay, J. (2021) Building collective control and improving health through a place-based community empowerment initiative: Qualitative evidence from communities seeking agency over their built environment. *Critical Public Health*, 31(3): 268–79. https://doi.org/10.1080/09581596.2020.1851654

Eke, O., Martin, A., Khidir, H., Otugo, O., Marshall, A., Suarez, J., and Konstantopoulos, W. (2021) Advocating for equity during the pandemic. *BMJ Leader*, 5. https://doi.org/10.1136/leader-2020-000380.

English, K. C., Fairbanks, J., Finster, C. E., Rafelito, A., Luna, J., and Kennedy, M. (2006) A socioecological approach to improving mammography rates in a tribal community. *Health Education and Behaviour*, 35: 396–409.

Epstein, S. (1996) *Impure science: AIDS, activism, and the politics of knowledge*. Berkeley: University of California Press.

Escobar, A. (1992) Imagining a post-development era? Critical thought, development and social movements. *Social Text*, (31/32): 20–56.

Esteva, G. and Prakash, M. S. (1998) Beyond Development, What? *Development in Practice*, 8(3): 280–96.

Etzioni, A. (1998) A communitarian note on stakeholder theory. *Business Ethics Quarterly*, 8(4): 679–91.

Everhart, K. (2012) Cultura–identidad: The use of art in the University of Puerto Rico student movement, 2010. *Humanity and Society*, 36(3): 198–219.

Fan, K. W. (2012) Schistosomiasis control and snail elimination in China. *American Journal of Public Health*, 102(12): 2231–2. https://doi.org/10.2105/AJPH.2012.300809

Farmer, P., Kim, J. Y., Kleinman, A., and Basilico, M. (2013) *Reimagining Global Health: An Introduction*. Berkeley: University of California Press.

Farrington, J., Bebbington, A., with Wellard, K., and Lewis, D. J. (1993) *Reluctant Partners: Non-governmental Organisations, the State and Sustainable Agricultural Development*. London: Routledge.

Fassin, D. (2003) The embodiment of inequality: AIDS as a social condition and the historical experience in South Africa. *EMBO Rep*, 4(1): S4–9. https://doi.org/10.1038/sj.embor.embor856

Fawcett, S. B., Collie-Akers, V., Schultz, J. A., and Cupertino, P. (2013) Community-based participatory research within the Latino health for all coalition. *Journal of Prevention and Intervention in the Community*, 41: 142–54.

Fehling, M., Nelson, B. D., and Venkatapuram, S. (2013) Limitations of the Millennium Development Goals: a literature review. *Global Public Health*, 8(10): 1109–22. https://doi.org/10.1080/17441692.2013.845676

Figueroa, J. P., Bottazzi, M. E., Hotez, P., Batista, C., Ergonul, O., Gilbert, S., ... and Kang, G. (2021) Urgent needs of low-income and middle-income countries for COVID-19 vaccines and therapeutics. *The Lancet*, 397(10274): 562–4.

Fiona, S., Maja, G., Carolin, H., and Miguel, N. (2011) Food, finance and fuel: the impacts of the triple F crisis in Nigeria, with a particular focus on women and children: Adamawa State Focus. *Overseas Development Institute, ODI*. Working paper. https://odi.org/en/publications/food-finance-and-fuel-the-impacts-of-the-triple-f-crisis-in-nigeria-with-a-particular-focus-on-women-and-children/

Fisher, M. (2003) Open mics and open minds: Spoken word poetry in African diaspora participatory literacy communities. *Harvard Educational Review*, 73(3): 362–89.

Flores, W. (2011) Community monitoring for accountability in health: review of literature. Open Society Foundations-Accountability and Monitoring in Health Initiative Public Health Program, 1–28.

Flores, W. and Samuel, J. (2019) Grassroots organisations and the sustainable development goals: No one left behind? *BMJ*, 365: l2269. https://doi.org/10.1136/bmj.l2269

Ford, L. (2017) Families, fertility and feminism: landmarks in women's rights. *The Guardian*, 17 July. https://www.theguardian.com/global-development/2017/jul/27/families-fertility-feminism-landmarks-in-womens-rights-timeline

Foucault, M. (1982) The subject and power. *Critical Inquiry*, 8(4): 777–95.

Fox, J. (2014) Social Accountability: What Does the Evidence Really Say? *Global Partnership for Social Accountability*. Working Paper No 1. https://documents1.worldbank.org/curated/en/964041607326557934/text/Social-Accountability-What-Does-the-Evidence-Really-Say.txt

Fox, J. and Robinson, R. (2023) Sandwich strategies explained: Expanding citizen action. MacArthur Foundation. http://www.macfound.org/press/perspectives/sandwich-strategies-explained-expanding-citizen-action

Freire, P. (1970) *Pedagogy of the Oppressed*. New York: Continuum.

Freire, P. (1973) *Education for Critical Consciousness*. New York: Continuum.

Freire, P. (1977) *Pedagogy in Process*. New York: Continuum.

Frontline World (2002) Bolivia – Leasing the rain timeline: Cochabamba water revolt, *PBS*. https://www.pbs.org/frontlineworld/stories/bolivia/timeline.html

Galbraith, J. K. (1954) Countervailing power. *The American Economic Review*, 44(2): 1–6.

Gatt, I., Raykov, M., and Vella, R. (2021) Not safe for work (NSFW): Persons living with HIV: A study of a socially engaged theatre work-in-progress. *Malta Review of Educational Research*, 15(S): 7–27.

Gaventa, G. (2002) Introduction: Exploring citizenship, participation and accountability. *IDS Bulletin*, 33(2): 1–11.

Gaventa, J. and McGee, R. (2013) The impact of transparency and accountability initiatives. *Development Policy Review*, 31: s3–s28. https://doi.org/10.1111/dpr.12017

Gavieta, M. (2020) The intersectionality of blackness and disability in hip-hop: The societal impact of changing cultural norms in music. *International Social Science Review*, 96(4): Article 2.

George, A. S., Mehra, V., Scott, K., and Sriram, V. (2015) Community participation in health systems research: A systematic review assessing the state of research, the nature of interventions involved and the features of engagement with communities. *PLoS ONE*, 10(10): e0141091.

Gergen, M. (2000) *Feminist Reconstructions in Psychology: Narrative, Gender, and Performance*. London: Sage Publications.

Germain, S. and Yong, A. (2020) COVID-19 Highlighting inequalities in access to healthcare in England: A case study of ethnic minority and migrant women. *Feminist Legal Studies*, 28: 301–10.

Ghai, A. and Johri, R. (2008) Prenatal diagnosis: Where do we draw the line? *Indian Journal of Gender Studies*, 15(2): 291–316.

Gilchrist, A. and Taylor, M. (2016) *The Short Guide to Community Development*. Bristol: Policy Press.

Gilmore, A., Fabbri, A., Baum, F., Bertscher, A., Bondy, K., and Chang, H.-J. (2023) Defining and conceptualising the commercial determinants of health. *Lancet*, 401(10383): 1194–213. https:// doi.org/10.1016/ S0140-6736(23)00013-2

Gilson, L. and Mills, A. (1995) Health sector reform in Sub Saharan Africa: Lessons of the last 10 years. *Health Policy*, 32(95): 215–43.

Glenn, C. L. (2015) Activism or "Slacktivism?": Digital media and organizing for social change. *Communication Teacher*, 29(2): 81–5. https://doi.org/ 10.1080/17404622.2014.1003310=

GoI – MoHFW (2005) National rural health mission: Meeting people's health needs in rural areas, framework of implementation 2005–12. http://mohfw.nic.in/NRHM/Community_monitoring/Implementers_ Manual.pdf

Good, C. M. (1991) Pioneer medical missions in Colonial Africa. *Social Science and Medicine*, 32(1): 1–10.

Goodheart, D. (2017) *Road to Somewhere: The Populist Revolt and the Future of Politics*. London: Hurst Publication.

Gonzalez, J. A. and McCarthy, D. (1999) *Bolivia - Public Expenditure Review (English)*. Washington, D.C.: World Bank Group. http://docume nts.worldbank.org/curated/en/689781468768283970/Bolivia-Public-Expenditure-Review

González-Agüero, M., Vargas, I., Campos, S., Cancino, A. F., Quezada, C., and Marchia, J. (2018) Lesbian, Gay, and Bisexual human rights as a global health issue. *Sociology Compass*, 12(12): e12642. https://doi.org/ 10.1111/soc4.12642

González-Agüero, M., Vargas, I., Campos, S., Farías Cancino, A., Quezada Quezada, C., and Urrutia Egaña, M. (2022) What makes a health movement successful? Health inequalities and the insulin pump in Chile. *Critical Public Health*, 32(2): 181–92. https://doi.org/10.1080/09581596.2020.1808190

Goodwin, J. and Jasper, J. M. (eds) (2003) *Rethinking Social Movements: Structure, Meaning, and Emotion*. Maryland: Rowman & Littlefield Publishers.

Goodwin, J. and Jasper, J. M. (eds) (2009) *The social movements reader: Cases and concepts* (No. 12). New York: John Wiley & Sons.

Graham, H. (2009) *Understanding Health Inequalities*. Maidenhead: McGraw-Hill; Open University Press.

Gramsci, A. (1971) Selections from the Prison Notebooks of Antonio Gramsci. Q. Hoare and G. N. Smith (eds) & (Trans.). New York: International Publishers.

Gumbonzvanda, N., Gumbonzvanda, F., and Burgess, R. (2021) Decolonising the 'safe space' as an African innovation: The Nhanga as quiet activism to improve women's health and wellbeing, *Critical Public Health*, 31(2): 169–81. https://doi.org/10.1080/09581596.2020.1866169

Guttman, N., Gesser-Edelsburg, A., and Aycheh, S. (2013) Communicating health rights to disadvantaged populations: Challenges in developing a culture-centered approach for Ethiopian immigrants in Israel, *Health Communication*, 28(6): 546–56. https://doi.org/10.1080/10410 236.2012.702643

Habermas, J. (1988) *On the logic of social sciences*. Cambridge, MA: MIT Press.

Habermas, J. (2008) New social movements. In V. Ruggiero and N. Montagna (eds) *Social Movements: A Reader*. London: Routledge, 201–5.

Haines, A., Sanders, D., Lehmann, U., Rowe, A. K., Lawn, J. E., Jan, S. et al (2007) Achieving child survival goals: Potential contribution of community health workers, *Lancet*, 369: 2121–31.

Haldane, V., Chuah, F. L., Srivastava, A., Singh, S. R., Koh, G. C., Seng, C. K., and Legido-Quigley, H. (2019) Community participation in health services development, implementation, and evaluation: A systematic review of empowerment, health, community, and process outcomes. *PLoS ONE*, 14(5): e0216112.

Hall, B. (1981) Participatory research, popular knowledge and power: A personal reflection. *Convergence*, 3: 6–19.

Halsall, T., Garinger, C., Dixon, K., and Forneris, T. (2019) Evaluation of a social media strategy to promote mental health literacy and help-seeking in youth. *Journal of Consumer Health on the Internet*, 23(1): 13–38. https://doi.org/10.1080/15398285.2019.1571301

Hamer, J. and Kapilashrami, A. (2020) Win-win collaboration? Understanding donor-private sector engagement in health and its implications for Universal Health Coverage. In J. Gideon, and E. Unterhalter (eds) *Critical Reflections on Public Private Partnerships*. London: Routledge, 214–33.

Hammonds, R. and Ooms, G. (2004) World Bank policies and the obligation of its members to respect, protect and fulfill the right to health. *Health and Human Rights*, 8(1): 26–60.

Hankivsky, O. and Kapilashrami, A. (2020) Intersectionality offers a radical rethinking of Covid-19. *BMJ Opinion Blog*, 15 May. https://blogs.bmj.com/bmj/2020/05/15/intersectionality-offers-a-radical-rethinking-of-covid-19/

Hardiman, M. (1986) People's involvement in health and medical care. In J. Midgley, with A. Hall, M. Hardiman, and D. Narine (eds) *Community Participation, Social Development and the State*. London: Methuen.

Harding, S. G. (1986) *The Science Question in Feminism*. Ithaca and London: Cornell University Press.

Harding, S. (1987) Introduction: Is there a feminist method? In S. Harding (ed) *Feminism and Methodology*. Bloomington: IUP, 1–14.

Harman, S. (2016) Bringing to life the reality of living as a woman with HIV/Aids in rural Tanzania. *The Conversation*. https://theconversation. com/bringing-to-life-the-reality-of-living-as-a-woman-with-hiv-aids-in-rural-tanzania-68680

Hartmann, H. I. and Markusen, A. R. (1980) Contemporary Marxist theory and practice: A feminist critique. *Review of Radical Political Economics*, 12(2): 87–94.

Healthwatch UP-Bihar (2001) *Priorities of the People: People Population Policies and Women's Health in Uttar Pradesh*. Lucknow: Sahayog.

Health Policy Watch (2024) 'Reverse the Reverse the Backsliding on Sexual and Reproductive Health and Rights: A Wake-up Call from Independent Scientists and Advisors'. Independent scientists and members of UN advisory groups. https://healthpolicy-watch.news/ reverse-the-backsliding-on-sexual-and-reproductive-health-and-rights/

Henderson, P. and Vercseg, I. (2010) *Community Development and Civil Society: Making Connections in the European Context*. Bristol: Policy Press, 97–106.

Heywood, M. (2009) South Africa's treatment action campaign: Combining law and social mobilization to realise right to health. *Journal of Human Rights Practice*, 1(1): 14–36.

Hickel, J. (2016) Neoliberalism and the end of democracy. In S. Springer, K. Birch, and J. MacLeavy (eds) *Handbook of neoliberalism*. London: Routledge, 142–52.

Hillery, G. A. (1955) Definitions of Community: Areas of Agreement. *Rural Sociology*, 20: 194–204.

Hoe, C., Weiger, C. R., Minosa, M. K., Alonso, F., Koon, A. D., and Cohen, J. E. (2022) Strategies to expand corporate autonomy by the tobacco, alcohol and sugar-sweetened beverage industry: A scoping review of reviews – Globalization and health. *BioMed Central*. https://globalizati onandhealth.biomedcentral.com/articles/10.1186/s12992-022-00811-x

Hoffmann, K. D. (2014) *The Role of Social Accountability in Improving Health Outcomes: Overview and Analysis of Selected International NGO Experiences to Advance the Field*. Washington, D.C.: CORE Group.

Holtz, A. (2007) Scriptdoctor: Medicine in the media: national survey shows Michael Moore's Sicko did indeed provoke discussions about US health care system. *Oncology Times*, 29(18): 28–9.

Hossain, S. M., Bhuiya, A., Khan, R., and Uhaa, I. (2004) Community development and its impact on health: South Asian experience. *BMJ*, 328: 830–3.

Hotez, P. J. (2021) *Preventing the Next Pandemic: Vaccine Diplomacy in a Time of Anti-science*. New York: Johns Hopkins University Press.

Howard-Jones, N. (1975) *The scientific background of the International Sanitary Conferences, 1851-1938*. Geneva: World Health Organization. https://iris. who.int/handle/10665/62873

HRBA Portal (2022) *The Human Rights Based Approach to Development Cooperation: Towards a Common Understanding of UN Agencies*. https://hrb aportal.org/the-human-rights-based-approach-to-development-cooperat ion-towards-a-common-understanding-among-un-agencies/

Hughto, J. M. W., Reisner, S. L., and Pachankis, J. E. (2015) Transgender stigma and health: A critical review of stigma determinants, mechanisms, and interventions. *Social Science & Medicine*, 147: 222–31. https://doi.org/ 10.1016/j.socscimed.2015.11.010

Hulac, B. (2016) Tobacco and oil industries used same researchers to sway public. *Scientific American*. https://www.scientificamerican.com/article/ tobacco-and-oil-industries-used-same-researchers-to-sway-public1/

Hunt, P. (2016) Interpreting the international right to health in a human rights-based approach to health. *Health and Human Rights*, 18(2): 109.

Hunyen, M. M. T. E., Martens, P., and Hilderink, H. B. M. (2005) The health impacts of globalisation: A Conceptual Framework. *Globalization and Health*, 1: 14. https://doi.org/10.1186/1744-8603-1-14

Hupe, P. and Hill, M. (2007) Street-level bureaucracy and public accountability. *Public Administration*, 85(2): 279–99.

Ife, J. W. (2013) *Community Development in an Uncertain World: Vision, Analysis and Practice*. Cambridge; Port Melbourne, Vic: Cambridge University Press.

Ife, J. and Fiske, L. (2006) Human rights and community work: Complementary theories and practices. *International Social Work*, 49(3): 297–308. https:// doi.org/10.1177/0020872806063403

Ikemire, H. (2010) Putting culture to work: building community with youth through community-based theater practice, Doctoral dissertation, Arizona State University.

Jain, R., Kelly, C. A., Mehta, S., Tolliver, D., Stewart, A., and Perdomo, J. (2021) A trainee-led social media advocacy campaign to address COVID-19 inequities. *Pediatrics*, 147(3): e2020028456. https://doi.org/10.1542/ peds.2020-028456

Jakarta (1996) Jakarta declaration. https://www.who.int/teams/health-promotion/enhanced-wellbeing/fourth-global-conference/jakarta-decl aration

Jocson, K. M. (2006) 'The best of both worlds': Youth poetry as social critique and form of empowerment. In S. Ginwright, P. Noguera, and J. Cammarota (eds) *Beyond Resistance! Youth Activism and Community Change: New Democratic Possibilities for Practice and Policy for America's Youth*. New York: Routledge, 129–47.

Joffe, C. E., Weitz, T. A., and Stacey, C. L. (2004) Uneasy allies: pro-choice physicians, feminist health activists and the struggle for abortion rights. *Sociology of Health & Illness*, 26(6): 775–96.

Johnson, B. (2020) *The history of quarantine and resistance to Public Health Measures.* https://nationalsecurityzone.medill.northwestern.edu/covid analyzer/news/the-history-of-quarantine-and-resistance-to-public-health-measures/

Joshi, A. and Houtzager, P. P. (2012) Widgets or watchdogs? Conceptual explorations in social accountability. *Public Management Review*, 14(2): 145–62.

Jurkowski, J. M. and Paul-Ward, A. (2007) Photovoice with vulnerable populations: Addressing disparities in health promotion among people with intellectual disabilities. *Health Promotion Practice*, 8(4): 358–65. https://doi.org/10.1177/1524839906292181

Kabeer, N. (2000) Resources, agency, achievements: Reflections on the measurement of women's empowerment. *Development and Change*, 30(3): 435–64.

Kantamaturapoj, K., Kulthanmanusorn, A., Witthayapipopsakul, W., Viriyathorn, S., Patcharanarumol, W., Kanchanachitra, C. et al (2020) Legislating for public accountability in universal health coverage, Thailand. *Bulletin of the World Health Organization*, 98: 117–25.

Kapilashrami, A. (2022) Intersectionality. In L. Monaghan and J. Gabe (eds) *Key Concepts in Medical Sociology*. London: Sage, 38–45.

Kapilashrami, A. and Baru, R. V. (eds) (2018) *Global Health Governance and Commercialisation of Public Health in India: Actors, Institutions and the Dialectics of Global and Local*. London: Routledge. https://doi.org/10.4324/978135 1049023

Kapilashrami, A. and Hankivsky, O. (2018) Intersectionality and why it matters to global health. *The Lancet*, 391(10140): 2589–91.

Kapilashrami, A. and Marsden, S. (2018) Examining intersectional inequalities in access to health (enabling) resources in disadvantaged communities in Scotland: advancing the participatory paradigm. *International Journal for Equity in Health*, 17(1): 83. https://doi.org/10.1186/s12939-018-0797-x

Kapilashrami, A. and McPake, B. (2013) Transforming governance or reinforcing hierarchies and competition: examining the public and hidden transcripts of the Global Fund and HIV in India. *Health Policy and Planning*, 28(6): 626–35. https://doi.org/10.1093/heapol/czs102

Kapilashrami, A. and O'Brien, O. (2012) The Global Fund and the re-configuration and re-emergence of 'civil society': Widening or closing the democratic deficit? *Global Public Health*, 7(5): 437–51.

Kapilashrami, A., Fustukian, S., and McPake, B. (2015) Global prescriptions and neglect of the 'local': What lessons for global health governance has the Framework Convention on Global Health learned? *Global Health Governance*, 9(1).

Kapilashrami, A., Smith, K. E., Fustukian, S., Eltanani, M. K., Laughlin, S., Robertson, T., ... and Scandrett, E. (2016) Social movements and public health advocacy in action: The UK people's health movement. *Journal of Public Health*, 38(3): 413–6.

Kapilashrami, A., Hill, S., and Meer, N. (2018) What can health inequalities researchers learn from an intersectionality perspective? Understanding social dynamics with an inter-categorical approach? *Social Theory & Health*, 13(3): 288–307.

Kasat, P. (2013) Community arts and cultural development: A powerful tool for social transformation. Masters' thesis, Murdoch University.

Kaur-Gill, S. (2022) The cultural customization of TikTok: subaltern migrant workers and their digital cultures. *Media International Australia*. https://doi.org/10.1177/1329878X221110279

Kentikelenis, A. E. (2017) Structural adjustment and health: A conceptual framework and evidence on pathways. *Social Science & Medicine*, 187: 296–305.

Keshet, Y. and Popper-Giveon, A. (2017) Neutrality in medicine and health professionals from ethnic minority groups: The case of Arab health professionals in Israel. *Social Science & Medicine*, 174: 35–42.

Khanday, Z. A. and Akram, M. (2012) Health status of marginalized groups in India. *International Journal of Applied Sociology*, 2(6): 60–70.

Khanna, R. and Pradhan, A. (2013) *Evaluation of the Process of Community Based Monitoring and Planning of Health Services in Maharashtra*. Pune: SATHI (Support for Advocacy and Training to Health Initiatives).

Kickbusch, I. (2015) The political determinants of health: 10 years on. *BMJ*, 350: h81. https://doi.org/10.1136/bmj.h81

Knight, M., Bunch, K., Vousden, N., Banerjee, A., Cox, P., Cross-Sudworth, F., ... and Kurinczuk, J. J. (2022) A national cohort study and confidential enquiry to investigate ethnic disparities in maternal mortality. *EClinicalMedicine*, 43: 101237.

Kreps, G. L. (2006) Communication and racial inequities in health care. *American Behavioral Scientist*, 49(6): 1–15.

Kretzmann, J. P. and McKnight, J. L. (1993) *Building communities from the inside out: A path toward finding and mobilizing a community's assets*. Chicago: ACTA Publications.

Kriesi, H. (1996) The organizational structure of new social movements in a political context. In D. McAdam, J. D. McCarthy, and M. N. Zald (eds) *Comparative perspectives on social movements*. Cambridge: Cambridge University Press, 152–84.

Kriesi, H., Koopmans, R., Duyvendak, J. W., and Giugni, M. G. (1992) New social movements and political opportunities in Western Europe. *European Journal of Political Research*, 22(2): 219–44.

Kropotkin, P. (1989) *Mutual Aid*. Montreal: Black Rose Books.

Labonté, R. and Ruckert, A. (2019) *Health Equity in a Globalizing Era: Past Challenges, Future Prospects*. Oxford: Oxford University Press.

Lagunju, A. and Papart, J. P. (2013) The Bamako Initiative: Wrong medicine for the wrong ailment. *Sahara Reporters*. https://www.tarsc.org/publications/documents/SOCEMP%20Framework%20TARSC%20final2016.pdf

Lassa, S., Saddiq, M., Owen, J., Burton, C., and Balen, J. (2022) Evolving power dynamics in global health: from biomedical hegemony to market dynamics in global health financing; a response to the recent commentaries. *International Journal of Health Policy and Management*, 12(1): 1–2.

Laverack, G. (2005) Power and empowerment. *Public Health: Power, Empowerment and Professional Practice*. London: Palgrave Macmillan, 27–36.

Laville, S. (2019) Top oil firms spending millions lobbying to block climate change policies, says report. *The Guardian*. http://www.theguardian.com/business/2019/mar/22/top-oil-firms-spending-millions-lobbying-to-block-climate-change-policies-says-report

Lawrence, F. (2019) Big Tobacco, war and politics. *Nature*. https://www.nature.com/articles/d41586-019-02991-w

Lawrence, M., Homer-Dixon, T., Janzwood, S., Rockstöm, J., Renn, O., and Donges, J. F. (2024) Global polycrisis: the causal mechanisms of crisis entanglement. *Global Sustainability*, 7: e6.

Lawson, D. W., Borgerhoff Mulder, M., Ghiselli, M. E., Ngadaya, E., Ngowi, B., Mfinanga, S. G., … and James, S. (2014) Ethnicity and child health in northern Tanzania: Maasai pastoralists are disadvantaged compared to neighbouring ethnic groups. *PLoS ONE*, 9(10): e110447.

Leal, A. P. (2007) Participation: The ascendancy of a buzzword in the neo-liberal era. *Development in Practice*, 17(4–5): 539–8.

Legge, D. G. and Kim, S. (2021) Equitable access to COVID-19 vaccines: Cooperation around research and production capacity is critical. *Journal for Peace and Nuclear Disarmament*, 4(sup1): 73–134.

Lehmann, U. and Sanders, D. (2007) *Community Health Workers: What Do We Know About Them?* Geneva: World Health Organization.

Lim, S. S., Dandona, L., Hoisington, J. A., James, S. L., Hogan, M. C., and Gakidou, E. (2010) India's Janani Suraksha Yojana, a conditional cash transfer programme to increase births in health facilities: An impact evaluation. *Lancet*, 375: 2009–23.

Lima, M. J. and Galea, S. (2018) Corporate practices and health: A framework and mechanisms. *Globalization and Health*, 14(1): 1–12.

Lindquist, A., Knight, M., and Kurinczuk, J. J. (2013) Variation in severe maternal morbidity according to socioeconomic position: A UK national case–control study. *BMJ Open*, 3(6): e002742.

Loewenson, R. (2000) Participation and accountability in health systems: The missing factor in equity. *Equinet Policy Series*, 9: 1–27.

Loewenson, R. (2016) Understanding and organising evidence on social power and participation in health systems. Training and Research Support Centre. https://www.tarsc.org/publications/documents/SOCEMP%20Framework%20TARSC%20final2016.pdf

Lofgren, H. (2004) Pharmaceuticals and the consumer movement: The ambivalences of 'patient power'. *Australian Health Review*, 28(2): 228–37.

Lukes, S. (2005) *Power: A Radical View*. Basingstoke: Palgrave Macmillan.

Maani, N., Collin, J., Friel, S., Gilmore, A. B., McCambridge, J., Robertson, L., and Petticrew, M. (2021) The need for a conceptual understanding of the macro and meso commercial determinants of health inequalities. *European Journal of Public Health*, 31(4): 674–5.

Maarse, H. (2006) Privatisation of healthcare in Europe: An eight country analysis. *Journal of Health Politics, Policy and Law*, 31(5).

Maguire, P. (1987) *Doing Participatory Research: A Feminist Approach*. Amherst: University of Massachusetts, Centre for International Education.

Mahon, M. (2000) The visible evidence of cultural producers. *Annual Review of Anthropology*, 29: 466–92.

Mamudu, H. M. and Glantz, S. A. (2009) Civil Society and the negotiation of the Framework Convention on Tobacco Control. *Global Public Health*, 4(2): 150–68

Mann, J. M. Gostin, L., Gruskin, S., Brennan, T., Lazzarini, Z., and Fineberg, H. V. (1994) Health and human rights. *Health Hum Rights*, 1(1): 6–23.

Mansuri, G. and Rao, V. (2013) *Localizing Development: Does Participation Work?* Policy Research Report. Washington, D.C.: World Bank.

Manton, J. and Gorsky, M. (2018) Health Planning in 1960's Africa: International Health Organisations and the Post Colonial State. *Med Hist*, 62(4): 425–48.

Marieskind, H. (1975) The Women's Health Movement. *International Journal of Health Services*, 5(2): 217–23. https://doi.org/10.2190/5XUN-VX3H-KMWM-F17M

Marmot, M. (2015) *The Health Gap*. London: Bloomsbury.

Marmot, M. and Wilkinson, R. (eds) (2005) *Social Determinants of Health*, 2nd edition. Oxford: Oxford Academic. https://doi.org/10.1093/acprof:oso/9780198565895.001.0001

Marmot, M., Friel, S., Bell, R., Houweling, T. A., and Taylor, S. (2008) Commission on Social Determinants of Health. Closing the gap in a generation: health equity through action on the social determinants of health. *Lancet*, 372(9650): 1661–9. https://doi.org/10.1016/S0140-6736(08)61690-6

Marshall, A. I., Kantamaturapoj, K., Kiewnin, K., Chotchoungchatchai, S., Patcharanarumol, W., and Tangcharoensathien, V. (2021) Participatory and responsive governance in universal health coverage: An analysis of legislative provisions in Thailand. *BMJ Global Health*, 6: e004117.

Martinez, M. G. and Kohler, J. C. (2016) Civil society participation in the health system: The case of Brazil's health councils. *Globalization and Health*, 12: 64. https://doi.org/10.1186/s12992-016-0197-1

Masih, N. (2022) A rare all-woman newsroom puts Indian documentary in contention for Oscar. *The Washington Post*. https://www.washingtonpost.com/world/2022/03/25/india-khabar-lahariya-oscars/

Massó-Guijarro, B., Pérez-García, P., and Cruz-González, C. (2021) Applied theatre as a strategy for intervention with disadvantaged groups: A qualitative synthesis. *Educational Research*, 63(3): 337–56.

Mayoux, L. (1995) Beyond naivety: Women, gender inequality and participatory development. *Development and Change*, 26(2): 235–58.

Mazza, N. (2007) Words from the heart: Poetry therapy and group work with the homeless. *Journal of Poetry Therapy*, 20(4): 203–9. https://doi.org/10.1080/08893670701714647

MBRRACE-UK (2022) Saving lives, improving mothers' care. Core report: Lessons learned to inform maternity care from the UK and Ireland confidential enquiries into maternal deaths and morbidity 2018–20. Oxford: MBRRACE-UK. National Perinatal Epidemiology Unit, University of Oxford. https://www.npeu.ox.ac.uk/assets/downloads/mbrrace-uk/reports/maternal-report-2022/MBRRACE-UK_Maternal_CORE_Report_2022_v10.pdf

McCarthy, D. (1996) *Knowledge as Culture: The New Sociology of Knowledge*. New York: Routledge.

McCarthy, J. D. and Zald, M. N. (1977) Resource mobilization and social movements: A partial theory. *American Journal of Sociology*, 82(6): 1212–41.

McCartney, G. (2011) Illustrating health inequalities in Glasgow. *Journal of Epidemiology & Community Health*, 65: 94.

McCoy, D. C., Hall, J. A., and Ridge, M. (2012) A systematic review of the literature for evidence on health facility committees in low-and middle-income countries. *Health Policy and Planning*, 27(6): 449–66.

McCoy, D., Kapilashrami, A., Kumar, R., Rhule, E., and Khosla, R. (2024) Developing an agenda for the decolonization of global health. *Bull World Health Organ*, 102(2): 130–6. https://doi.org/10.2471/BLT.23.289949

McCowan, T. (2023) Landless Workers Movement. *Encyclopedia Britannica*. https://www.britannica.com/event/Landless-Workers-Movement

McGee, R. and Gaventa, J. (2011) Shifting power? Assessing the impact of transparency and accountability initiatives. *IDS Working Papers*, 383: 1–39.

Mendenhall, E. (2017) Syndemics: a new path for global health research. *The Lancet*, 389(10072): 889–91.

Minkler, M., Rebanal, R. D., Pearce, R., and Acosta, M. (2019) Growing equity and health equity in perilous times: Lessons from community organizers. *Health Education & Behavior*, 46(1_suppl): 9S–18S. https://doi.org/10.1177/1090198119852995

Mishra, P. (2017) *The Age of Anger*. London: Picador.

Misra, U. (2021) Explainspeaking: What 2020 taught us about India's internal migration. *Indian Express*. https://indianexpress.com/article/explained/what-2020-taught-us-about-indias-internal-migration-explainspeaking-7189053/

Mitton, C., Smith, N., Peacock, S., Evoy, B., and Abelson, J. (2011) Integrating public input into healthcare priority-setting decisions. *Evidence & Policy*, 7(3): 327–43.

Mohan, G. and Stokke, K. (2000) Participatory development and empowerment: The dangers of localism. *Third World Quarterly*, 21(2): 247–68.

Mohan, G. (2007) Participatory development: From epistemiological reversals to active citizenship. *Geography Compass*, 1(4): 779–96. https://doi.org/10.1111/j.1749-8198.2007.00038.x

Molyneux, S., Atela, M., Angwenyi, V., and Goodman, C. (2012) Community accountability at peripheral health facilities: A review of the empirical literature and development of a conceptual framework. *Health Policy and Planning*, 27(7): 541–54.

Mona, H., Andersson, L. M., Hjern, A., and Ascher, H. (2021) Barriers to accessing health care among undocumented migrants in Sweden – A principal component analysis. *BMC Health Services Research*, 21(830). https://doi.org/10.1186/s12913-021-06837-y

Moorhead, S. A., Hazlett, D. E., Harrison, L., Carroll, J. K., Irwin, A., and Hoving, C. (2013) A new dimension of health care: Systematic review of the uses, benefits, and limitations of social media for health communication. *Journal of Medical Internet Research*, 15(4): e85.

Mosse, D. (2001) 'People's knowledge', participation and patronage: operations and representations in rural development. In B. Cooke and U. Kothari (eds) *Participation: The New Tyranny?* London: Zed Press, 16–35.

Moussa, M. B. (2013) From arab street to social movements: Re-theorizing collective action and the role of social media in the Arab Spring. Westminster papers in Communication and Culture, Arab Media and Society. *Canadian Journal of Communication and Stream: Culture and Technology*, 9(2).

Mulreany, J. P., Calikoglu, S., Ruiz, S., and Sapsin, J. W. (2006) Water privatization and public health in Latin America. *Rev Panam Salud Publica*, 19(1): 23–32.

Mulumba, M., London, L., Nantaba, J., and Ngwena, C. (2018) Using health committees to promote community participation as a social determinant of the right to health: Lessons from Uganda and South Africa. *Health and Human Rights*, 20(2): 11.

Musolino, C., Baum, F., Freeman, T., Labonté, R., Bodini, C., and Sanders, D. (2020) Global health activists' lessons on building social movements for Health for All. *International Journal for Equity in Health*, 19(1): 1–14.

Nair, Y. and Campbell, C. (2008) Building partnerships to support community-led HIV/AIDS management: a case study from rural South Africa. *African Journal of AIDS Research*, 7(1): 45–53.

Nair, M., Kurinczuk, J. J., and Knight, M. (2014) Ethnic variations in severe maternal morbidity in the UK–a case control study. *PLoS ONE*, 9(4): e95086.

Nampoothiri, N. J. and Artuso, F. (2021) Civil society's response to coronavirus disease 2019: Patterns from two hundred case studies of emergent agency. *Journal of Creative Communications*, 16(2): 203–12. https://doi.org/10.1177/09732586211015057

Nandi, S., Vracar, A., and Pachhauli, C. (2020) Resisting privatisation and marketisation of healthcare: People's Health Movement's experiences from India, Philippines and Europe, *Saúde Debate*, 44: 37–50.

Narayan, R. (2006) The role of the People's Health Movement in putting the social determinants of health on the global agenda. *Health Promotion Journal of Australia*, 17(3): 186–8.

Narayan, R. and Schuftan, C. (2004) The People's Health movement: A people's campaign for "Health for All-Now!". *Perspectives on Global Development and Technology*, 3: 235–43. https://doi.org/10.1163/1569150042036611

Nasir, R. (2014) Muslim self exclusion and public health services in Delhi. *South Asia Review*, 34(1): 65–86.

National Academy of Medicine (n.d.) Achieving health equity and systems transformation through community engagement: A conceptual model. https://nam.edu/programs/value-science-driven-health-care/achieving-health-equity-and-systems-transformation-through-community-engagement-a-conceptual-model/

National Campaign Against Torture (NCAT) (2020) Police brutality & unwarranted deaths dent India's covid-19 lockdown National Campaign Against Torture. http://www.uncat.org/banner/police-brutality-unwarranted-deaths-covid-19-lockdown/

NDTV (2021) Only two child policy can remove poverty among Assam Muslims: Himanta Biswa Sarma, *NDTV*, 29 July. https://www.ndtv.com/india-news/only-2-child-policy-can-remove-poverty-among-assam-muslims-himanta-biswa-sarma-2475510

Newell, K. W. (1975) *Health by the People*. Geneva: World Health Organization.

Newell, P. (2006) Corporate Accountability and Citizen Action: Companies and Communities in India. In R. Mohanty and R. Tandon (eds) *Participatory Citizenship: Identity, Exclusion, Inclusion*. New Dehli: Sage Publications.

Nikkhah, H. A. and Redzuan, M. (2009) Participation as a medium of empowerment in community development. *European Journal of Social Sciences*, 11(1): 170–6.

Nisbet, R. A. (1953) *The Quest for Community: A Study in the Ethics of Order and Freedom*. New York: Oxford University Press.

Nizar, S. (2016) *The Contradiction in Disability Law: Selective Abortions and Rights*. New Dehli: Oxford University Press.

Norris, T. and Pittman, M. (2000) The healthy communities movement and the coalition for healthier cities and communities. *Public Health*, 115(2–3): 118–24.

Nunn, A., Fonseca, E. D., and Gruskin, S. (2009) Changing global essential medicines norms to improve access to AIDS treatment: Lessons from Brazil. *Global Public Health*, 4(2): 131–49. https://doi.org/10.1080/1744169080 2684067

Nutbeam, D. (2008) The evolving concept of health literacy. *Social Science & Medicine*, 67: 2072–8.

Nyonator, F. K., Awoonor-Williams, J. K., Phillips, J. F., Jones, T. C., and Miller, R. A. (2005) The Ghana community-based health planning and services initiative for scaling up service delivery innovation. *Health Policy Plan*, 20(1): 5–34. https://doi.org/10.1093/heapol/czi003

Oakley, P. (1995) *People's Participation in Development Projects* (Vol. 7). Oxford: Intrac.

Office of the High Commissioner of Human Rights (n.d.) Gender Equality and Gender Backlash. https://www.ohchr.org/sites/default/files/Docume nts/Issues/Women/WG/Gender-equality-and-gender-backlash.pdf

OHCHR (2020) 'States responses to Covid 19 thread should not halt freedoms of assembly and association': UN expert on the rights to freedoms of peaceful assembly and of association, Mr Clement Voule. https://www. ohchr.org/en/statements/2020/04/states-responses-covid-19-threat-sho uld-not-halt-freedoms-assembly-and??

OHCHR (2000) CESCR General Comment No. 14: The Right to the Highest Attainable Standard of Health (Art. 12). Geneva: Office of the United Nations High Commissioner for Human Rights. https://www. ohchr.org/sites/default/files/Documents/Issues/Women/WRGS/Health/ GC14.pdf

Oliveira Cruz, V. and McPake, B. (2011) Global Health Initiatives and aid effectiveness: insights from a Ugandan case study. *Globalization and Health*, 7: 1–10.

Osaghae, E. E., Favareto, A., Mohanty, R., Piper, L. E., Mahmud, S., Waldman, L., ... and Ruiz, C. C. (2010) *Citizenship and Social Movements: Perspectives from the Global South*. London: Bloomsbury Publishing.

Ottersen, O. P., Dasgupta, J., Blovin, C., Buss, P., Chongsuvivatwong, V., Frenk, J., et al (2014) The Lancet – University of Oslo commission on global governance for health: the political origins of health inequity: prospects for change. *The Lancet*, 383: 630–67. https://doi.org/10.1016/ S0140-6736(13)62407-1

Ottowa (1986) https://www.who.int/teams/health-promotion/enhanced- wellbeing/first-global-conference

Papp, S. A., Gogoi, A., and Campbell, C. (2013) Improving maternal health through social accountability: A case study from Orissa, India. *Global Public Health*, 8(4): 449–64.

Parfitt, T. (2004) The ambiguity of participation: A qualified defence of participatory development. *Third World Quarterly*, 25(3): 537–55.

Pearce, J. (2020) Remembering COVID: Past epidemics and history lessons of the future. https://pushkin-house.squarespace.com/blog/2020/9/3/bob nqjo4c379lohyyr7go22ka6qhh3

Perry, H. B. and Rohde, J. (2019) The Jamkhed Comprehensive Rural Health Project and the Alma-Ata Vision of Primary Health Care. *American Journal of Public Health*, 109(5): 699–704. https://doi.org/10.2105/AJPH.2019.304968

Peruzzotti, E., Smulovitz, C., Arato, A. Behrend, J., Calvancanti, R. B., Fuentes, C. A., Grau, N. C., Lemos-Nelson, A. T., O'Donnell, G., Rivera, A. J. O., Peruzzotti, E., Przeworski, A., Smulovitz, C., Waisbord, S. R., and Zaverucha, J. (2006) Social accountability: An introduction. In E. Peruzzotti and C. Smulovitz (eds) *Enforcing the Rule of Law: Social Accountability in the New Latin American Democracies*. Pittsburg, PA: University of Pittsburgh Press, 3–33. https://doi.org/10.2307/j.ctt9qh5t1.6

Petersen, A., Schermuly, A. C., and Anderson, A. (2019) The shifting politics of patient activism: From bio-sociality to bio-digital citizenship. *Health*, 23(4): 478–94.

Pfeiffer, J. and Chapman, R. (2010) Anthropological perspectives on structural adjustment and public health. *Annual Review of Anthropology*, 39: 149–65.

Phillips, H. (2014) The return of the Pholela experiment: Medical history and primary health care in post-Apartheid South Africa. *American Journal of Public Health*, 104(10): 1872–6. https://doi.org/10.2105/AJPH.2014.302136

PHM (2021) PHM Policy Brief Unpacking the Covax Black Box, June. https://phmovement.org/wp-content/uploads/2021/08/Final-policy-brief-Covax_compressed_English.pdf

Pichardo, N. A. (1997) New social movements: A critical review. *Annual Review of Sociology*, 23(1): 411–30.

Pilkington, V., Keestra, S. M., and Hill, A. (2022) Global COVID-19 Vaccine Inequity: Failures in the First Year of Distribution and Potential Solutions for the Future. *Frontiers in Public Health,* 10: 821117. https://doi.org/10.3389/fpubh.2022.821117

Popple, K. (2015) *Analysing Community Work: Theory and Practice.* Maidenhead, Berkshire: McGraw-Hill Education.

Potash, S. (2011) Movie to Movement: Creating Social Change with the Documentary Film 'Food Stamped'. https://digitalrepository.unm.edu/educ_hess_etds/62

Proudhon, P. J. (1979) *The Principle of Federation*. Toronto: University of Toronto Press.

Poudrier, J. and Mac-Lean, R. T. (2009) 'We've fallen into the cracks': Aboriginal women's experiences with breast cancer through photovoice. *Nursing Inquiry*, 16(4): 306–17. https://doi.org/10.1111/j.1440-1800.2009.00435.x

Prasad, B. M. and Muraleedharan, V. R. (2007) *Community Health Workers: A Review of Concepts, Practice and Policy Concerns*. London: International Consortium for Research on Equitable Health Systems (CREHS).

Pretty, J. N. (1995) *A Trainer's Guide for Participatory Learning and Action*. London: IIED.

Purcell, R. (2007) Images for change: Community development, community arts and photography. *Community Development Journal*, 44(1): 111–21.

Putnam, R. D. (1993) The prosperous community: Social capital and public life. *The American Prospect*, 4(13): 35–42.

Quinn, N., Shulman, A., Knifton, L., and Byrne, P. (2011) The impact of a national mental health arts and film festival on stigma and recovery. *Acta Psychiatrica Scandinavica*, 123(1): 71–81. https://doi.org/10.1111/j.1600-0447.2010.01573.x

Rahman, M. A. (1993) *People's self development*. London: Zed.

Rahman, F. (2018) Working with Muslims: Beyond Burqa and Triple Talaq review: Life on the Margins. *The Hindu*, July 14. https://www.thehindu.com/books/books-reviews/working-with-muslims-beyond-burqa-and-triple-talaq-review-life-on-the-margins/article24410395.%E2%80%A6

Rahnema, M. (1992) Participation. In W. Sachs (ed) *The Development Dictionary: a guide to knowledge as power*. London: Zed Press, 116–31.

Raksin, A. (1987) Silent spring Rachel Carson. *Los Angeles Times*. https://www.latimes.com/archives/la-xpm-1987-10-25-bk-16150-story.html

Ramakant Rai v. Union of India (2003) W.P (C) No 209 https://www.casemine.com/judgement/in/581180bc2713e179479c7cbd

Ramirez, A. G., Aguilar, R. P., Merck, A., Despres, C., Sukumaran, P., Cantu-Pawlik, S., and Chalela, P. (2021) Use of #SaludTues Tweetchats for the dissemination of culturally relevant information on Latino health equity: exploratory case study. *JMIR Public Health and Surveillance*, 7(3): e21266. https://doi.org/10.2196/21266

Ramos, C. (2021) Beyond the Columbian exchange: Medicine and public health. *Colonial Latin America History Compass*, 19: e12682. https://doi.org/10.1111/hic3.12682

Rao, M. (2004) *From Population Control to Reproductive Health: Malthusian Arithmetic*. New Delhi: SAGE.

Rappaport, J. (1984) Studies in empowerment: Introduction to the issue. *Prevention in Human Services*, 3: 1–7.

Rashid, O. (2020) Coronavirus: In Bareilly, migrants returning home sprayed with 'disinfectant'. *The Hindu.* https://www.thehindu.com/news/national/other-states/coronavirus-in-bareilly-migrants-forced-to-take-bath-in-the-open-with-sanitiser/article61956440.ece

Ravallion, M. (1997) Can high inequality countries escape absolute poverty? *Economic Letters*, 56(1): 51–57.

Ravindran, S. (2014) Poverty, food security and universal access to sexual and reproductive health services: A call for cross-movement activism against neoliberal globalization. *Reproductive Health Matters*, 22(43): 14–27.

Rege, S. (1998) Dalit women talk differently: A critique of 'difference' and towards a Dalit feminist standpoint position. *Economic and Political Weekly*, 33(44): 39–46.

Reid, C. (2004) Advancing Women's Social Justice Agendas: A Feminist Action Research Framework. *International Journal of Qualitative Methods*, 3(3): 1–15. https://doi.org/10.1177/160940690400300301

Reuters (2021) More than 40,000 march in Vienna against coronavirus lockdown. https://www.reuters.com/world/europe/thousands-march-vienna-against-coronavirus-lockdown-2021-12-04/

Ribera-Almandoz, O. and Clua-Losada, M. (2021) Health movements in the age of austerity: rescaling resistance in Spain and the United Kingdom. *Critical Public Health*, 31(2): 182–92. https://doi.org/10.1080/09581596.2020.1856333

Rickard, E. and Ozieranski, P. (2021) A hidden web of policy influence: The pharmaceutical industry's engagement with UK's All-Party Parliamentary Groups. *PLoS ONE*, 16(6): e0252551.

Rifkin, S. B. (1996) Paradigms lost: Toward a new understanding of community participation in health programmes. *Acta Tropica*, 61(2): 79–92.

Rifkin, S. B. (2009) Lessons from community participation in health programmes: a review of the post Alma-Ata experience. *International Health*, 1(1): 31–36.

Riggs, E., Davis, E., Gibbs, L., Block, K., Szwarc, J., Casey, S. et al (2012) Accessing maternal and child health services in Melbourne, Australia: Reflections from refugee families and service providers. *BMC Health Services Research*, 12: 117.

Ritterbusch, A. E. (2016) Exploring social inclusion strategies for public health research and practice: The use of participatory visual methods to counter stigmas surrounding street-based substance abuse in Colombia. *Global Public Health*, 11(5–6): 600–17.

Robinson, D. (2022) 10 companies called out for greenwashing. https://earth.org/greenwashing-companies-corporations/

Robson, S. and Spence, J. (2011) The erosion of feminist self and identity in community development theory and practice. *Community Development Journal*, 46(3): 288–301.

Rodriguez, S. (2013) Making sense of social change: Observing collective action in networked cultures. *Sociology Compass*, 7(12): 1053–64.

Ruault, L. and Rundell, E. (2016) The transnational circulation of feminist self-help: The second act in the fight for abortion rights? *Critique internationale*, 70: 37–54.

Ruger, J. (2007) Global health governance and the World Bank. *Lancet*. 370(9597): 1471–4. https://doi.org/10.1016/S0140-6736(07)61619-5

Rushton, S. (2023) Women's Cooperatives overcome water wars and climate drought in Rojava. https://www.equaltimes.org/women-s-cooperatives-overcome?lang=en

Ruthven, J. S. (2016) 'Making it personal': Ideology, the arts, and shifting registers in health promotion. *AIDS Care*, 28(4): 72–82. https://doi.org/10.1080/09540121.2016.1195485

Saini, A. (2016) Physicians of colonial India (1757–1900). *Journal of Family Medicine and Primary Care*, 5: 528–32.

Samuel, J., Flores, W., and Frisancho, A. (2020) Social exclusion and universal health coverage: Health care rights and citizen-led accountability in Guatemala and Peru. *International Journal for Equity in Health*, 19(1): 1–9.

Samuels, F., Gavrilovic, M., Harper, C., and Nino-Zarazua, M. (2011) Food, fuel and finance: the impacts of the triple F crisis on women and children-Adamawa State focus. Overseas Development Institute. Working Paper. https://cdn.odi.org/media/documents/7395.pdf

Sapra, I. and Nayak, B. P. (2021) The protracted exodus of migrants from Hyderabad in the time of COVID-19. *Journal of Social and Economic Development*, 23(2): 398–413. https://doi.org/10.1007/s40847-021-00155-z

SATHI (2010) *Compiled Report of the Community Based Monitoring of Health Services in Maharashtra (2007–10)*. Pune: SATHI. http://www.sathicehat.org/uploads/CurrentProjects/CBM_Report_June10_Final.pdf

Schmid, H., Bar, M., and Nirel, R. (2008) Advocacy activities in nonprofit human service organizations: Implications for policy. *Nonprofit and Voluntary Sector Quarterly*, 37(4): 581–602.

Seda, O. and Chivandikwa, N. (2014) Power dynamics in applied theatre: Interrogating the power of the university-based TfD facilitator – the UZ theatre and CARE Zimbabwe's Zvishavane/Mberengwa NICA project and SSFP as case study. *Research in Drama Education: The Journal of Applied Theatre and Performance*, 19(2): 143–58.

Sekoni, A. O., Jolly, K., and Gale, N. K. (2022) Hidden healthcare populations: Using intersectionality to theorise the experiences of LGBT+ people in Nigeria, Africa. *Global Public Health*, 17(1): 134–49. https://doi.org/10.1080/17441692.2020.1849351

Sen, A. (1999) *Development as Freedom*. New York: Oxford University Press.

Seow, H., McMillan, K., Civak, M., Bainbridge, D., van der Wal, A., Haanstra, C. et al (2021) #Caremongering: A community-led social movement to address health and social needs during COVID-19. *PLoS ONE*, 16(1): e0245483. https://doi.org/10.1371/journal.pone.0245483

Shaeffer, P. (2008) New thinking on poverty: Implications for globalisation and poverty reduction strategies DESA Working Paper No 65 ST/ESA/2008/DWP/65

Shalev, C., Kaplan, G., and Guttman, N. 2006. Public knowledge about health rights according to the law: What does the public know? In G. Gur and G. Bin-Nun (eds) *A Decade to the Israel National Health Insurance Law.* Tel Hashomer, Israel: The Israel Health Policy Institute, 501–7.

Sheikh, A. (2006) Why are ethnic minorities under-represented in US research studies? *PLoS Med*, 3: e49.

Shukla, A., Saha, S., and Jadhav, N. (2013) *Community Based Monitoring and Planning in Maharashtra: A Case Study.* Pune, India: SATHI and COPASAH.

Silva, A. S., De Sousa, M. S. A., Da Silva, E. V., and Galato, D. (2019) Social participation in the health technology incorporation process into Unified Health System. *Revista de Saude Publica.* https://doi.org/10.11606/S1518-8787.2019053001420

Simon-Kumar, R. (2017) Who is marginalised? Conflicting accounts of disadvantage in policy engagement. *Women's Studies Journal*, 31(1).

Singh, P. (2021) Populism, nationalism, and nationalist populism. *St Comp Int Dev*, 56: 250–69. https://doi.org/10.1007/s12116-021-09337-6

Siyech, M. S. and Jouhar, N. (2020) Civil society and Covid 19 in India: Unassuming heroes. Middle East Institute. https://www.mei.edu/publications/civil-society-and-covid-19-india-unassuming-heroes

Sjollema, S. and Hanley, J. (2014) When words arrive: a qualitative study of poetry as a community development tool. *Community Development Journal*, 49(1): 54–68.

Smith, M. F. and Ferguson, D. P. (2010) Activism 2.0. In R. L. Heath (ed) *The SAGE handbook of public relations.* Thousand Oaks, CA: Sage, 395–407.

Smith, B. G., Krishna, A., and Al-Sinan, R. (2019) Beyond Slacktivism: Examining the Entanglement between Social Media Engagement, Empowerment, and Participation in Activism. *International Journal of Strategic Communication*, 13(3): 182–96. https://doi.org/10.1080/1553118X.2019.1621870

Solar, O. and Irwin, A. (2010) A conceptual framework for action on the social determinants of health. Social determinants of health discussion paper 2 (Policy and Practice). Geneva: World Health Organization.

Springer, S., Birch, K., and MacLeavy, J. (eds) (2016) *Handbook of Neoliberalism.* New York: Routledge. https://doi.org/10.4324/9781315730660

Stephney, P. and Popple, K. (2008) *Social Work and the Community: A Critical Context for Practice.* Basingstoke: Palgrave Macmillan.

Stern, T. (2019) Participatory action research and the challenges of knowledge democracy. *Educational Action Research*, 27(3): 435–51.

Sumriddetchkajorn, K., Shimazaki, K., Ono, T., Kusaba, T., Sato, K., and Kobayashi, N. (2019) Universal health coverage and primary care, Thailand. *Bull World Health Organ*, 97(6): 415–22. https://doi.org/10.2471/BLT.18.223693

Supran, G. and Oreskes, N. (2021) Rhetoric and frame analysis of ExxonMobil's climate change communications. *One Earth*, 4(5): 696–719. https://doi.org/10.1016/j.oneear.2021.04.014

Tandon, R. (1988) Social transformation and participatory research. *Convergence*, 21(2): 5–18.

Tandon, T. (1996) The historical roots and contemporary tendencies in participatory research: Implications for health care. In K. De Koning and M. Martin (eds) *Participatory Research in Health: Issues and Experiences*, 2nd edition. London: Zed Books, 19–26.

Tandon, R. and Aravind, R. (2021) *Source of Life or Kiss of Death*: Revisiting state–civil society dynamics in India during COVID-19 pandemic. *Nonprofit Policy Forum*, 12(1): 147–63. https://doi.org/10.1515/npf-2020-0045

Tangcharoensathien, V., Tisayaticom, K., Suphanchaimat, R. Vongmongkol, V., Viriyathorn, S., and Limwattananon, S. (2020) Financial risk protection of Thailand's universal health coverage: Results from series of national household surveys between 1996 and 2015. *Int J Equity Health*, 19(163). https://doi.org/10.1186/s12939-020-01273-6

Tanne, J. (2007) US health professionals demonstrate in support of Sicko. *BMJ: British Medical Journal*, 334(7608): 1338.

Tarrow, S. G. (1993) *Power in Movement: Social Movements, Collective Action, and Mass Politics in the Modern State*. Cambridge: Cambridge University Press.

Tarrow, S. G. (2011) *Power in Movement: Social Movements, Collective Action, and Mass Politics in the Modern State*, 2nd edition. Cambridge: Cambridge University Press.

Taylor, C.E. (1956) Country doctor in India. *The Atlantic* (June 1956 issue). https://www.theatlantic.com/magazine/archive/1956/06/country-doctor-in-india/642915/

Taylor-Gooby, P. and Stoker, G. (2011) The Coalition Programme: A New Vision for Britain or Politics as Usual? *The Political Quarterly*, 82(1): 4–15.

The Lancet. (2020) COVID-19: Remaking the social contract. *The Lancet*, 395: 1401. https://doi.org/10.1016/s0140-6736(20)30983-1

The Hindu (2021) UP's new Population Policy keeps all sections in mind: Adityanath. https://www.thehindu.com/news/national/ups-new-population-policy-keeps-all-sections-in-mind-adityanath/article35263976.ece

The Indian Express (2021) Survivors of Bhopal Gas tragedy launch 37-day campaign seeking justice. https://indianexpress.com/article/cities/bhopal/bhopal-gas-tragedy-survivors-campaign-37th-anniversary-7591551/

The Tribune (2006) Nitish has big plans for 'resurgent Bihar'. *The Tribune*, 8 November. https://www.tribuneindia.com/2006/20061209/nation.htm#4

Theocharis, Y., Lowe, W., van Deth, J. W., and García-Albacete, G. (2015) Using twitter to mobilize protest action: Online mobilization patterns and action repertoires in the occupy wall street, indignados, and aganaktismenoi movements. *Information, Communication & Society*, 18(2): 202–20. https://doi.org/10.1080/1369118X.2014.948035

Thompson, L. and Tapscott, C. (2010) *Citizenship and Social Movements: Perspectives from the Global South.* London: Zed Books.

Thompson, E. E. and Ofori-Parku, S. S. (2021) Advocacy and mobilizing for health policy change: Ghanaian news media's framing of a prescription opioid crisis. *Health Communication*, 36(14): 1909–20. https://doi.org/10.1080/10410236.2020.1808403

Thomson, M., Kentikelenis, A., and Stubbs, T. (2017) Structural adjustment programmes adversely affect vulnerable populations: a systematic-narrative review of their effect on child and maternal health. *Public Health Reviews*, 38(1): 1–18.

Tilly, C. (1977) Studying social movements/studying collective action. CRSO Working paper #168. University of Michigan. https://deepblue.lib.umich.edu/bitstream/handle/2027.42/50943/168.pdf

Tobin, J. (2012) *The Right to Health in International Law.* Oxford: Oxford University Press.

Tognotti, E. (2013) Lessons from the history of quarantine, from plague to influenza A. *Emerg Infect Dis*, 19(2): 254–9. https://doi.org/10.3201/eid1902.120312

Tollman, S. (1991) Community oriented primary care: Origins, evolution, applications. *Soc Sci Med*, 32(6): 633–42.

Tönnies, F. (2001) *Tönnies: Community and Civil Society.* M. Hollis (trans.) and J. Harris (ed). Cambridge: Cambridge University Press.

Tuckman, B. W. (1965) Developmental sequence in small groups. *Psychological Bulletin*, 63(6): 384.

Tufte, T. and Mefalopulos, P. (2009) *Participatory Communication: A Practical Guide* (Vol. 170). Washington, D.C.: World Bank Publications.

Twelvetrees, A. (1991). What is Community Work? In *Community Work. Practical Social Work.* London: Palgrave. https://doi.org/10.1007/978-1-349-21262-0_1

United Nations Economic and Social Council (1984). *Siracusa Principles on the Limitation and Derogation of Provisions in the International Covenant on Civil and Political Rights.* Paris: United Nations Commission on Human Rights.

Van Belle, S., Boydell, V., George, A. S., Brinkerhof, D. W., and Khosla, R. (2018) Broadening understanding of accountability ecosystems in sexual and reproductive health and rights: A systematic review. *PLoS ONE*, 13(5): e0196788.

Van Buren, K. (2011) Music, HIV/AIDS and Social Change in Nairobi, Kenya. In G. Barz and J. Cohen (eds) *The Culture of AIDS in Africa: Hope and Healing through Music and the Arts*. New York: Oxford University Press, 70–84.

Van Stekelenburg, J. and Klandermans, B. (2009) Social movement theory: past, present and prospects by. In *Movers and shakers. Social Movements in Africa*, 17–43. http://www.mendeley.com/research/social-movement-theory-past-present-prospects-4

Vélez-Vélez, R. and Villarrubia-Mendoza, J. (2019) Interpreting mobilization dynamics through art: A look at the DREAMers Movement. *Current Sociology*, 67(1): 100–21. https://doi.org/10.1177/0011392118807517

Vikram, K., Sharma, A. K., and Kannan, A. T. (2013) Beneficiary level factors influencing Janani Suraksha Yojana utilization in urban slum population of trans-Yamuna area of Delhi. *The Indian Journal of Medical Research*, 138(3): 340–6.

Visaria, L., Acharya, A., and Raj, F. (2006) Two child norm: Victimising the vulnerable. *EPW*, 41(01). https://www.epw.in/journal/2006/01/spec ial-articles/two-child-norm.html

Wade, L. (2020) An unequal blow. *Science*, 368(6492): 700–3.

Wadman, M. (1999) Gore under fire in controversy over South Africa AIDS drug law. *Nature*, 399: 717–8. https://doi.org/10.1038/21472

Wallerstein, N. (1999) Power between evaluator and community: Research relationship within New Mexico's healthier communities. *Social Science & Medicine*, 49(1): 39–53.

Wallerstein, N. (2006) *What Is the Evidence on Effectiveness of Empowerment to Improve Health?* Copenhagen: WHO Europe, Health Evidence Network.

Wallerstein, N., Duran, B. M., Aguilar, J., Joe, L., Loretto, F., Toya, A., … and Shendo, K. (2003) Jemez Pueblo: Built and social-cultural environments and health within a rural American Indian community in the Southwest. *American Journal of Public Health*, 93(9): 1517–8.

Wang, C. C. (2003) Using Photovoice as a participatory assessment and issue selection tool: A case study with the homeless in Ann Arbor. In M. Minkler and N. Wallerstein (eds) *Community-based Participatory Research for Health*. San Francisco: Jossey-Bass, 180–96.

Wang, C. C. and Burris, M. A. (1997) Photovoice: Concept, methodology, and use for participatory needs assessment. *Health Education & Behavior*, 24(3): 369–87.

Weale, A., Kieslich, K., Littlejohns, P., Tugendhaft, A., Tumilty, E., Weerasuriya, K., and Whitty, J. A. (2016) Introduction: Priority setting, equitable access and public involvement in health care. *Journal of Health Organization and Management*, 30(5): 736–50. https://doi.org/10.1108/JHOM-03-2016-0036

Werner, D. and Bower, B. (1982) *Helping Health Workers Learn*. Berkeley, CA: Hesperian Health Guides.

Werner, D., Thuman, C., and Maxwell, J. (1992) *Where there is no doctor : a village health care handbook* (Rev. ed). Berkeley, CA: Hesperian Foundation.

White, S. C. (1996) Depoliticising development: The uses and abuses of participation. *Development in Practice*, 6(1): 6–15.

WHO (1978) Declaration of Alma-Ata. International Conference on Primary Health Care. Alma-Ata, USSR, 6–12 September, paras. III, VII5.

WHO (1986) Ottawa Charter for Health Promotion World Health Organisation. Geneva: World Health Organization.

WHO (2018) Declaration of Astana. Global Conference on Primary Health Care. Astana, Kazakhstan, 25–26 October. Geneva: World Health Organization.

WHO (2023) WHO celebrates the role of communities in driving progress towards ending AIDS, WHO News release. https://www.who.int/news/item/29-11-2023-who-celebrates-the-role-of-communities-in-driving-progress-towards-ending-aids

WHO (2024a) Social participation for universal health coverage, health and well-being. https://apps.who.int/gb/ebwha/pdf_files/WHA77/A77_R2-en.pdf

WHO (2024b) Commercial determinants of noncommunicable diseases in the WHO European region. World Health Organization, Regional Office for Europe. https://iris.who.int/handle/10665/376957

Wiktorowicz, Q. (2004) *Islamic Activism: A Social Movement Theory Approach.* Bloomington, IN: Indiana University Press.

Wilkinson, R. and Pickett, K. (2010) *The Spirit Level: Why Equality Is Better for Everyone.* London: Penguin.

Wilson, E. (1980) *Only Halfway to Paradise: Women in Postwar Britain, 1945-1968.* London: Tavistock Publications.

World Bank (1989) *Sub-Saharan Africa: From crisis to sustainable development.* Washington, D.C.: World Bank.

World Bank (2001) *World Development Report 2000/2001: Attacking Poverty. World Development Report.* New York: Oxford University Press. https://openknowledge.worldbank.org/handle/10986/11856

Worsley, P. (1967) *The Third World.* Chicago: University of Chicago Press.

Wrentschur, M. and Moser, M. (2014) 'Stop: Now we are speaking!' A creative and dissident approach of empowering disadvantaged young people. *International Social Work*, 57(4): 398–410. https://doi.org/10.1177/0020872814526764

Young, M. D. and Wilmott, P. (1957) *Family and Kinship in East London.* London: Routledge.

Index

Note: References to figures appear in *italic* type.

Bhore Committee report (1946) 28, 35
Big Lottery initiative 37
'Big Society' flagship policy programme
  (2010) 11
Bill and Melinda Gates Foundation
  (BMGF) 114
bio-digital citizenship 99, 169
Black Death (plague) 146
#BlackLivesMatter movement 60, 155, 170
bodily autonomy 4, 42, 91, 100
#bombadeinsulinaalAUGE movement 170
Bono (singer), Make Poverty History
  campaign 109
Brazil 37–8
  citizens' media, journalism in 167–8
  Movimento dos Trabalhadores Rurais Sem
    Terra, land reforms movements in 48, 182
  Sistema Unico de Saude (Unified Health
    System) 38, 43, 130
  social participation 130
  and US pharma industry 110, 113
breast cancer movement 79–80, 93, 99
Bretton Woods 11
Brexit 44, 121
Brigadista Populares, Nicaragua 35
Brussels, COVID-19 protests 145

C

Canada 118, 155
  Aboriginal women health, and
    photovoice 79–80
  and arts as community development
    tool 164
  Caremongering movement 171
#CancelTheDebt campaign 108
capacity building 55, 61, 94, 127, 132, 178
CEDAW 130
Chile
  #bombadeinsulinaalAUGE in 170
  social media and health advocacy in 170
China 7, 34, 150, 166
  barefoot doctors 35
  LGBTQ awareness in 163
  mass health programmes 28
  poverty reduction in 107
  Queer Comrades 162, 163
Chipko movement, against
  deforestation 64
Cholera 31, 32–3, 147
citizen action 126, 137–8
citizen participation 11, 38, 61,
  133, 135–6
CIVICUS report 145
civil rights movements 10, 61, 84, 155,
  160–1, 170
civil society 8–9, 18, 41, 47, 55–6, 99,
  125, 126, 127, 157
  against tobacco use 112

and accountability 130, 131
and advocacy 58, 96–7, 149–53, 156
in Arab countries 87
bureaucratisation of 97
during COVID-19 pandemic 144, 147
fragmentation of action spaces 96
and state, relationship between 64–5
climate action 118, 120
climate change 10, 109, 115, 116–20, *117*
CO₂ Coalition 118
Coalition for Epidemic Preparedness and
  Innovations (CEPI) 114
Cochabamba Water War, in Bolivia 25,
  102–3, 104
collective action 3, 21–2, 26, 49, 53,
  55, 59–60, 75, 85–8, 96, 127, 157,
  167, 183
collectivising, social media communities
  in 169–70
colonisation 6–7, 11–12, 13, 14, 31–2, 55,
  62, 64, 160
Colombia, photography 162, 165
Columbus, Christopher 29–31
Combahee River Collective 57
commercialisation
  commercial determinants of health
    (CDoH) 24, 103, 110–15, 121, 124
  Commercial Healthcare Distribution
    Market 112
  commercial interests, in public policy in
    health systems 98–9, 137
communal demography 152–3
communitarianism 46, 58, 60
community development 6–7, 9, *45*,
  55–6, 81, 94
  arts within 158–66
  in (post)colonial world 62–5
  pre-colonial histories of 11
  and theoretical ideas 56–60
  in Western Europe and North
    America 61–2
Community Health Workers
  (CHWs) 81
Community of Practitioners on
  Accountability and Social Action in
  Health (COPASAH) 132, 176
community participation/engagement 11,
  12, 18–20, 33, 39, *40*, 48–51, 74–6,
  133, 137, 175, 177–8
  affecting health service 37–40
  community health in 33–7
  framework for progressive realisation
    (Kapilashrami) 39–40, *40*
  in health, frameworks for 19–22
  in healthcare, history of 28–33, *34*
  in identity and discrimination 42
  and neoliberal wave 42–3
  NGOs 41–2